YOGA THERAPY FOR AUTOIMMUNE DISEASES

HOW TO MANAGE INFLAMMATION AND PAIN
WITH YOGA, RELAXATION AND MEDITATION

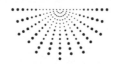

LILIANE NAJM

CONTENTS

INTRODUCTION

Did you know that autoimmune diseases are common, affecting over 23 million Americans and 2 million Canadians? They are a leading cause of death and disability especially among women. Some autoimmune diseases are rare, while others like hypothyroid disease affect many people.

Yoga therapy uses well-defined yoga postures in a sequence together with pranayama (breathing techniques) to help maintain and heal the body. It can help reduce symptoms associated with some ailments by the regular practice of a simple flow of yoga poses in a sequence to bring the body to maximum good health.

WHAT IS YOGA THERAPY?

A SAFE AND regular practice of yoga therapy can:

- decrease stress
- relieve anxiety
- reduce inflammation
- improve heart health
- improves the quality of life
- fight depression
- reduce chronic pain
- reduce menopausal symptoms
- promote sleep quality
- improves flexibility, balance, and mobility in older people
- help improve breathing
- relieve migraines
- promote healthy eating habits, and
- increase strength.

The International Association of Yoga Therapy says even if all "yoga is potentially therapeutic and healing, yoga therapy is the specific application of yogic tools—postures/exercises, breath work, meditation techniques, and more—to address an individual's physical, mental, and emotional needs."

Yoga therapy is complementary to Western or Chinese medicine. Complementary therapies are usually used alongside the more standard medical care. They view health and disease different from western medicine, which is starting to look at patients in a more holistic way. Yoga therapy has its basis in Ayurveda. The way it is mostly practiced in the western world is not related to a specific religion or sect but as a system to healing and good health.

Yoga therapists receive a rigorous training to help them test you and keep you, their client, safe. They are trained to work one-on-one with individuals and do not take the place of doctors, chiropractors, or physical therapists. They are motivated to teach individuals how the mind, body and prana work experientially, and take limitations into consideration. They will give you customized practices that include movements, breathing techniques, meditation and/or visualization, as well as physical poses that take care of specific areas of discomfort or musculoskeletal imbalances.

The advantage of yoga therapy over mainstream yoga is that it pays special attention to the individual. It is about people, not conditions. Working with clients as individuals is important as individuals require different practices to help you manage their condition(s).

The focus in yoga therapy is on synchronizing movement with the breath, stretching muscles that are tight and strengthening muscles that are weak. Yoga therapy deals mostly with chronic pain.

Your first session with a qualified yoga therapist will be an intake to find out your medical history and assess where your body is out of balance. Based on these findings, a yoga practice sequence is recommended. It is helpful to continue seeing a yoga therapist on a regular basis as the recommended sequence may change depending on your state of health and wellbeing.

WHAT IS AN AUTOIMMUNE DISEASE?

AN AUTOIMMUNE DISEASE is a condition where your immune system erroneously attacks your body. The immune system inaccurately think that some parts of the body are external and releases antibodies that attack healthy cells. They are the medical equivalent of friendly fire, and can cause serious damage.

The immune system is the body's defense against infectious organisms and other external invaders. When it becomes underactive or overactive, it is usually due to an immune system disease. If the immune system is overactive, the body attacks and damages its own tissues. If the immune system is underactive, the body's ability to fight invaders causing vulnerability to infections is diminished.

Overall, autoimmune diseases are common, affecting more than 23 million Americans and about 2 million Canadians. Yoga therapy, relaxation and meditation are useful.

Annex 1 at the end of this book has a short description of some of the autoimmune diseases.

THE KOSHIC MODEL OR
FRAMEWORK OF THE HUMAN BODY,
MIND, AND SPIRIT

YOGA THERAPY USES a model based on the koshas – a yogic illustration of a person's anatomy. The koshas are the distinct layers of a person. They give a full explanation and design a strategy to become healthy and complete. The koshic model comes to us from an ancient science of the mind called Vedanta, and is helpful in understanding how yoga poses work to get a greater understanding of ourselves.

Ayurveda is the basis for this model. It aims to manage and unite body, mind, and spirit using an interconnected approach by giving special importance to diet, herbal remedies, yoga, breathing techniques, and meditation.

The koshas are a model to explain the different facets that make us human. The word kosha means "sheath" or "level". In the koshic model, the goal of yoga therapy is to bring the koshas into balance. If one kosha is out of balance, it can influence the other koshas unsuitably. Yoga therapists test koshic imbalances and teach personalized practices to balance them.

Having a yoga therapist lead you into a yoga session is ideal, but you are still better off knowing more about yoga therapy and what goes on in a yoga therapy session. Learning gives you the ability to direct or influence your behaviour and perhaps the course of events.

KOSHAS OR LAYERS OF AWARENESS

OUR BODY IS FORMED of many-sided sheaths of matter of different depths surrounding and pervading a small physical core. Five sheaths or bodies are located in roughly the same place but in different dimensions. They range from gross to fine starting with the Annamayakosha or "foodstuff" sheath; Pranamayakosha or the "energy" sheath; Manomayakosha or the "mind-stuff" sheath; Vijnanamayakosha or the "wisdom" sheath; and finally Anandamayakosha or the "bliss" sheath.

These five layers of awareness serve as a guide to understand our energy bodies. They have distinct areas of activity but are in fact unified in approaching health and healing. They are one, and we and the world are part of this Unity. The koshas are not in any order of importance and do not have to be worked with separately.

Disease is separation at one koshic level or another. Yoginis and yogis believe that separation from our spiritual source is at the root of all issues and problems.

Here are details of the field of activity of each, its connection to health, and how yoga poses help in creating balance in each and in relation to each other moving us to good health. I have included in this book some yoga postures with a note on their valued influence on some conditions.

Annamayakosha or the Physical Body–the five elements of earth, water, fire, air, and space link to bring balance in the physical systems. These elements are balanced through an understanding of the Ayurvedic doshas (explained below). Yoga poses are essential for balancing the physical body and the doshas.

Pranamayakosha or the Energy Body—made of prana, the vital body force that holds the body and the mind together. This level connects to the subtle energy systems of the body, including the energy centers called chakras and the energy currents called Vayus. This level relates to balance in the energy centers and the flow of prana through us. Energy comes from Prana that gives life to all of creation. Illness can occur when prana is obstructed. Yoga poses open the energy channels.

Manomayakosha or the Psycho-Emotional Body/Mental Body—made of the mind. This is about the vital drives and the emotional responses associated with them such as the fight-or-flight response, survival and reproduction, and social roles. Obstruction in this body shows first as stress then as physical or mental disease. Yoga poses are the main vehicle for relieving stress and promoting relaxation.

Vijnanamayakosha or the Wisdom Body/Intuition Body—made of the intellect, the faculty that determines. This level is discerning wisdom and intuition, and the capacity to recognise patterns of living that are physically unhealthy and emotionally troubling. It is at this level that we notice patterns and eventually transform them. Yoga poses bring the calm concentration that is indispensable for the body.

Anandamayakosha or the Bliss Body—this is the true self. The nature of the Self is directed in thought and action by one's own values rather than external norms of happiness. Experiencing this level is temporary, but as we become more mindful of our true nature, we understand that we are complete at each moment. Yoga poses assist in realizing this true self.

Understanding the koshic model helps the yoga therapist to design practices that benefit all the aspects of the person. Individual yoga sessions with a qualified yoga therapist increase awareness and integration through the koshas, starting with the physical body leading to self-knowledge and to good health.

ELEMENTS

I TALKED EARLIER about the five elements and the three doshas. In Ayurveda, the five elements are the blocks of matter, life, and of our physical bodies. The features of each element are:

Earth—this element is the base from which life emanates. It is solid and connects to the physical body.

Water—this element is adaptable and penetrating. It connects to the energy body.

Fire—this is the element of energy, sunlight, willpower, and transformation. It connects to the psycho-emotional body.

Air—this element is about subtlety, movement, communication, speed and upward movement. It connects to the wisdom body.

Ether—this element is about spirit, causation, inner space (thoughts, imagery, dreams, attitude, and feelings) and outer space (external environment). It connects to the bliss body.

According to Vedanta, which is one of the six schools of Hindu philosophy, the sage knows of the influences of the five elements within each kosha and realizes the Self in its different aspects.

DOSHAS OR ARCHETYPES OF PHYSICAL BODIES

THE DOSHAS ARE a typical example of a person related to the five elements. Each person has a dominant dosha or a combination of doshas. Ayurvedic medicine considers that health is achieved through balancing the three doshas.

Vata—a combination of air and space. When Vata is out of balance, movement and instability can lead to poor digestion, insomnia and psychological problems.

Pitta—the element is mostly fire with some water. Pitta relates to the digestive power necessary for metabolism. When Pitta is out of balance, digestive problems and ulcers can result.

Kapha—a combination of earth and water. When Kapha is out of balance, congestion and respiratory problems may occur.

Annex 2 takes you through one of the practices to bring the doshas back into balance.

PRANA VAYUS ("WIND, BREATH, OR LIFE FORCE")

PRANA IS the universal creative energy and the energy that circulates in the body and manages bodily functions to operate properly. In yoga, this arrangement of fundamental vitality works through five sub-energies called the prana vayus. Each vayu has a unique job. If we grasp the part that each prana vayu plays, we can get a handle on how prana serves the person and how aggravations between the pranas lead to diminished satisfaction.

Prana takes five forms or vayus; each vayu has its own body area and main health functions.

Udana Vayu—situated in the throat and head, its energy moves in a clockwise circular motion. It regulates thought, communication, the senses, and the nervous system. Inconsistency in this area leads to problems of cognition and communication.

Prana Vayu— situated in the heart, chest, and lungs, it has an upward movement of energy responsible for breathing and circulation. Inconsistency here can lead to heart and lung conditions.

Samana Vayu— situated in the abdomen, it expands the abdominal area on inhalation and relaxes it on exhalation and is associated with the digestive fire. Inconsistency here can affect the digestive organ.

Apana Vayu— situated below the navel, we experience its energy as a downward flowing movement on the exhalation. It is responsible for downward movement of energy and produces elimination. Inconsistency here might lead to menstrual problems, sexual dysfunction, and constipation.

Vyana Vayu—directs the prana from the core body out to the extremities. It is associated with the peripheral nervous system and circulation, and distribution of energy that comes from food. Inconsistency here can lead to poor fringe circulation.

CHAKRAS OR WHEELS OF ENERGY

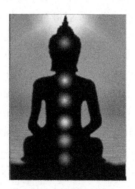

CHAKRAS ARE vital energy centers responsible for balance at all levels of our being. They are wheels of energy along the spine. Yoga poses were developed to open and balance the chakras. Appreciating the relationship between the chakras and the poses is necessary to get the benefits of the poses. Each chakra opens a different aspect of our being and can be energized by one or more pose categories.

The vayus are in the chakras. When a Vayu is off balance, the chakra associated with it will be affected unfavourably.

Health is affected by any disruption between the five vayus and their wheels of energy.

The seven main chakras are:

Muladhara chakra—positioned at the base of the spine, its element is earth, and its color is red. It relates to the Annamayakosha. When imbalanced, it deals with issues of survival, but when balanced it means groundedness and safety. Standing poses are beneficial.

Healing practices recommended for this chakra are movements to reconnect with the body; exercise and physical activity; massage and grounding work.

Swadhisthana chakra—can be found four fingers below the navel, its element is water and its color is orange. It relates to the Pranamayakosha. When imbalanced, it deals with issues of intimacy and emotions, but when balanced it means a healthy sexuality. Hip opening and stabilizing poses are beneficial.

Healing practices recommended for this chakra are mindful movement; emotional release; healthy pleasures; and work on finding boundaries.

Manipura chakra—situated in the solar plexus, its element is fire and its color is yellow. It relates to the Manomayakosha. When imbalanced it deals with issues of self-esteem and social roles, but when balanced it means healthy social roles. Twist poses are beneficial.

Healing practices recommended for this chakra are

stress management and deep relaxation; vigorous exercise; psychotherapy; and emotional connection.

Anahata chakra—to be found in the heart center, its element is air and its color is green. It relates to the Manomayakosha/Vijnanamayakosha. When imbalanced it deals with issues of depression and pessimism, but when balanced it is unconditional love. Back bend and lateral bend poses are beneficial.

Healing practices recommended for this chakra are breathing techniques; work with arms reaching in and out; journal writing; and psychotherapy.

Vishuddha chakra—located in the throat, its element is space and its color is blue. It relates to the Vijnanamayakosha. When imbalanced it deals with issues of communication, but when balanced it is internally directed Self. Forward bend poses are beneficial.

Healing practices recommended for this chakra are loosening the neck and shoulders; singing and chanting; storytelling and journal writing; creativity and psychotherapy.

Ajna chakra—positioned in the area between the eyebrows in what is called in yoga as the third eye. It has all the elements and its color is violet. It is related to the Anandamayakosha. When imbalanced it deals with issues of dedication to spiritual life, but when balanced it calms and sharpens focus. Balancing poses are beneficial.

Healing practices recommended for this chakra are visual arts and stimulation and meditation.

Sahasrara (the thousand-petal lotus) chakra—positioned in the crown of the head, its element is thought and its color is violet or crystal light. It relates to the Anandamayakosha. When imbalanced it deals with issues of spiritual separation, but when balanced it is Unity consciousness. Inverted poses are beneficial.

Healing practices recommended for this chakra are learning and study; meditation; psychotherapy; and re-establishing physical, emotional and spiritual connection.

BANDHAS OR ENERGETIC LOCKS

THE BANDHAS ARE energetic locks performed during yoga poses to direct the flow of energy in the body to bring about the benefits of the pose.

The three main bandhas are:

Mulabandha—situated at the perineum, is engaged by gently pulling the pelvic floor up into the body. If we imagine the body as a vessel with energy inflowing and leaving, we can intensify the energy in the body by locking the bottom of the vessel with this bandha. Mulabandha supports yoga practice by giving a strong foundation in strengthening the abdominal floor.

Uddiyanabandha—situated in the abdomen, is engaged by gently pulling the abdominal wall back toward the spine and up. If we imagine the body as a vessel of energy, we can seal its sides and control the energy within it. Uddiyanabandha can help prevent disc injuries in yoga practice by strongly supporting the abdomen, waist and low back.

Jalandharabandha—situated at the throat, is engaged by gently bringing the chin close to the sternum to seal the energy between the torso and the head. This way, we seal the top of the vessel of energy. In inverted yoga poses, we stop excessive energy from moving up into the head. We usually combine this bandha with the other two.

MUDRAS OR HANDS GESTURES

MUDRA MEANS "GESTURE". Yoga mudras are gestures practiced mostly with the hands and fingers. They facilitate the flow of energy in the subtle body.

Different yoga mudras bring different benefits. Mudras are often part of a yoga class. Different areas of the hands relate to different areas in the body and the brain. When we place our hands in yoga mudras, we stimulate different areas of the brain and create a specific energy circuit in the body. By doing this, we help generate a specific state of mind.

Anjali mudra also called Namaste/Prayer gesture is perhaps the most well-known mudra. This gesture shows that you love and honor yourself and the universe. Yogis use it at the start and the end of yoga practice while saying the word Namaste which means peace.

Here is a description of some mudras that are helpful for some conditions.

- For hypothyroidism and tension in the neck and

shoulders – Gently press the tips or pads of the thumbs until you sense the best energetic connection. The other fingers gently curl or extend out. It is believed that this mudra balances the thymus, thyroid and pituitary glands, and opens the throat, neck and upper lungs.

- For fear, anxiety, a wandering mind and stress conditions – Join the thumb to the index finger and extend the other three. Sense the energy in the circle formed by the thumb and index fingers. Let the palm of the hand be a reservoir of this energy. It is believed that this mudra balances all the physical systems of the body and centers the mind.

- For overall health and level of energy – Gently press together the tips or pads of all fingers until you can sense the best energetic connections. Perform this mudra for 5 to 10 breaths.

- For immune imbalance and heart disease – Place the hands together in front of the heart, and keep a small empty space between the palms. Feel the contact between the fingers and at the base of the palms. Keep the forearms parallel to the earth without forcing. It is believed that this mudra is beneficial for all physical systems and has a calming effect on the mind.

GUNAS OR ARCHETYPES OF MENTAL STATES

THE GUNAS ARE energies in the natural world and in the mind. They reveal the opposite properties in nature with an active energy, a static energy, and a balance energy. All activities in nature are aspects of the gunas and their constantly changing patterns. In us, these changes are our difficulties, mood swings, and fluctuating outlooks. Yoga makes us aware of the gunas to become free from their control.

> *Rajas*—the energy of activity, change, evolution, and development. In the mind, it is the energy of attachment, wanting, and desire. It is the drive to hunt and get food by overpowering and winning. Rajas is the fight aspect of the "fight-or-flight" response.

> *Tamas*—inertia or lack of movement. In the mind, it is a resistance to change, apathy or a feeling of being 'stuck'. It is also the shadow side of our nature, emotions that are dormant and repressed. Tamas represents another aspect of the "fight-or-flight" response that is the freeze response.

Sattva—between rajas and tamas. In the mind, sattva is clarity and light. It is peace, balance and harmony between rajas and tamas.

LANGHANA/BRAHMANA OR
ENERGETIC PRINCIPLES

THE PRACTICE of yoga creates a state of balance, reducing both the extremes of rajas and tamas and promoting the state of sattva. To secure this balance, it is important to understand what poses are appropriate for balancing different states of the body and mind. The Ayurvedic principle of Langhana and Brahmana allows us to understand the relative effects of the poses from relaxing to energizing.

Yoga poses and pranayama or breathing techniques are divided into two energetic principles: Brahmana and Langhana.

> *Langhana* means to lessen. It refers to yoga practices that slow metabolism, relax the nervous system, cool the body and ease the mind. These practices are helpful when rajas overcomes the body and mind, as they help rid your system of excess.

> *Brahmana* means to grow. It refers to yoga practices that increase metabolism, energize the nervous system, heat the body, and stimulate the mind. These practices are helpful

when tamas overcomes the body and mind and when your system is weak, as they build energy.

By balancing rajas and tamas with the regular and safe practice of yoga poses as they relate to the notion of Langhana and Brahmana, we can reach the sattvic state, which is the way to know our own self above the three gunas.

Let's now move to the topic of inflammation.

INFLAMMATION AND PAIN

INFLAMMATION IS a defensive method used by the body's immune system in different situations to counter and remove foreign bodies. It can be a reaction to a surgical procedure, infection, foreign body, or a substance that causes an allergic reaction. It can be due to unhealthy diets, food allergies, chronic infections, stress, tiredness, and an inactive lifestyle. Inflammation is a source of pain.

Pain is a common experience for people and shows that something is wrong. Pain can be either acute or chronic.

A sharp pain that starts without warning and lasts for a short time, no more than three months, is acute pain. It means something is wrong and needs assessment. It could be caused by burns or cuts, injuries, and infections. Some of its signs are anxiety, nausea, vomiting, hypertension, rapid heartbeat, perspiring, shallow respiration, restlessness, and the functional weakness as we grow older.

Pain because of harm to muscles, ligaments and tendons in the body is normal. It can lead to meaningless physical, psychological, and emotional suffering. Inadequate pain relief could cause declined immunity, infections, increased illness, and increased risk of developing chronic pain.

Chronic pain, such as back pain, joint pain, or shingles, is pain that lasts over six months. Frequently, it means reduced mobility, the incapability to care for oneself, anxiety, and social isolation. It negatively impact the quality of our life.

Individuals with autoimmune diseases sometimes follow advice to take substances to suppress symptoms instead of treating the disease itself, like when they take over-the-counter pills to suppress a sore throat. It is important to understand the symptoms as they help us to discover the real development of the disease. We can help our body to heal by treating the advance of the disease instead of suppressing symptoms. We must find out why are we sick, not only what disease do we have.

HOW CAN YOGA THERAPY HELP KEEP CHRONIC INFLAMMATION IN CHECK?

REGULAR MIND-BODY PRACTICES of yoga and meditation have a positive impact on the general health of the person. The regularity of the practice under the guidance of a qualified yoga therapist is essential.

Besides medications and self-care prevention, mindfulness meditation can help lessen pain, reduce anxiety, and improve the quality of our life. Meditation is an effective therapy that is simple, inexpensive, and can be used whenever and wherever you wish.

Several studies show that a regular safe practice of yoga lowers stress hormones that generate inflammation. The practice of yoga reduces inflammation, which is helpful in arthritic conditions, and relieves severe pain seen in diseases like fibromyalgia.

Yoga is an amazing method to fight stress and encourage healthy habits in body and mind. Many people practice yoga and/or meditation typically to reduce stress, and research back them up. When we reduce our stress levels, we help to reduce inflammation in our body and increase our well-being.

A regular and safe yoga practice increases an anti-inflammatory hormone. If you are suffering from adrenal fatigue and feel aches and pain, difficulty in sleeping or digestive problems, practice yoga and meditation as they are useful in keeping your parasympathetic nervous system under control. The parasympathetic nervous system functions to decrease blood pressure and heart rate and create a relaxation response. Breathing deeply and mindfully helps to improve the functioning of the parasympathetic nervous system.

Remember to listen to your body, rest when you need to, and adjust or stop if something is painful. By managing your body intuitively, you will help to avoid not only inflammation but many other physical and mental issues. Trust Your Intuition. Muscle assessment, done by the yoga therapist, is a great way to learn to listen to and trust your intuition. It is a fact that our thoughts and emotions directly affect our health.

As you use yoga to strengthen and heal your mind and body, you will find increased clarity, hope, strength and confidence. Adding yoga to your weekly routine, together with eating healthy food, and taking it easy when needed, can help reduce inflammation to a great degree. I know this from personal experience.

The medical world believes that chronic inflammation generate other chronic diseases like diabetes, thyroid issues, arthritis, and poor weight management. If we embrace suitable lifestyle choices, we will be able to positively influence the levels of inflammation in our bodies.

In January 2014, the OHIO State University led a research

study on how Yoga Can Lower Fatigue, Inflammation in Breast Cancer Survivors. They found that practicing yoga for as little as three months can reduce fatigue and lower inflammation. They also found that even a modest practice over several months could have significant benefits. The research focused on women with breast cancer, but the head of the research team believes that results could include people who are dealing with fatigue and inflammation. Yoga has many parts to it—stretching and strengthening, breathing, visualizing, and meditating. The researchers believe that the breathing and meditation components are important in seeing favorable changes.

Dr. Baxter Bell, MD, says that if we already live a healthy lifestyle it does not mean that we are immune to the effect of low level inflammation. But doing yoga and meditating on a regular basis will help us to effectively manage usual stress, and we know that stress and trauma play a big role in causing or worsening inflammation.

AN ANTI-INFLAMMATORY YOGA SEQUENCE

THIS IS a simple yoga practice to help reduce inflammation by relieving muscle aches and enhancing circulation and respiration. Your body becomes better able to fight stress, and will function in a way that improves circulation and breathing. These yoga poses also improve the digestive health that connects to your immune system response and inflammation.

Practice yoga in the morning and/or evening for ten minutes or more. Let time pass between eating and doing yoga. Let your attention be on your breathing as you move through a pose or hold it. As you continue to practice, you can increase the time you hold each pose within reasonable limits. It is important that you work within your own range of limits and abilities.

How to Practice:

Cat-Cow-Child flow–Repeat 6 to 12 times. Each breath consists of one inhale and one exhale.

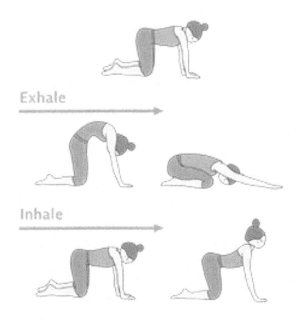

Exhale

Inhale

Caution:

People with neck injuries should keep the head in line with the torso and avoid dropping it forward or back.

Pregnant women and those with back injuries do only the Cow Pose, bringing the spine back to neutral between poses while avoiding to let the belly drop between repetitions, as this can strain the lower back.

If you have any medical concerns, talk with your doctor before you start this practice.

Benefits:

Cat-Cow-Child is a gentle flow of three poses that warms the body and brings flexibility to the spine. It stretches the back, torso, and neck. It carefully tones and strengthens the abdominal organs, and brings the spine into correct alignment. It opens the chest, encouraging the breath to become slow and deep. When you coordinate this movement with your breathing, you will help to calm the mind.

- Table pose – Come on your hands and knees with your wrists directly under your shoulders, and your knees directly under your hips. Point your fingertips to the top of your mat or thick blanket. Let your shins and knees be away from each other about hip-width apart. Center your head in a neutral position and soften your gaze downward.
- Cat pose – As you exhale, draw your belly to your spine and round your back toward the ceiling. The pose looks like a cat stretching its back. Release the crown of your head toward the floor, but don't force your chin to your chest.
- Cow pose – Inhale as you drop your belly towards the mat or blanket. Lift your chin and chest and look forward or up. Widen across your shoulder blades and take your shoulders away from your ears.
- Child pose – Rest back on your heels and place your arms by your sides or stretched forward and rest the forehead on the floor or on a prop. Press your pelvis back on their heels and lengthen the spine forward. Make sure that your shoulders are down away from your ears, stretch your hands gently back and turn the palms up or stretch them in front of you.

- Breathe in when you come back into Cow pose and breathe out as you return to Cat pose.
- Repeat 6 to 12 times and then rest by sitting back on your heels with your torso upright.

Mountain Pose (Standing Well) – Breathe normally and hold the pose for 5 breaths. Each breath consists of one inhale and one exhale.

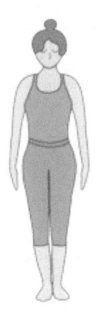

Caution:

Avoid the Mountain pose if you have a headache, insomnia, low blood pressure, or if you feel lightheaded.

Benefits:

A correctly done Mountain pose will use every muscle in the body. It improves posture and can help reduce back pain when you practice it regularly.

It strengthens the thighs, knees, ankles, abdomen, and buttocks. It is helpful to relieve sciatica pain.

It brings a calm focus. Practicing the pose with a steady and smooth breath will help relieve stress and improve concentration.

- Stand with your feet together and your arms at your sides. Gently press your weight evenly on the floor. Breathe steadily and rhythmically. Direct your attention inward and focus on the present moment, letting go of worries and concerns.
- Press lightly your big toes together (separate your heels if you need to). Lift your toes and spread them apart. Then, place them back down on the mat.
- If you have trouble balancing, stand with your feet six inches apart (about 15 cm) or wider, or place a hand on a wall or a chair for support.
- Ground your feet firmly into the earth. Then, lift your ankles and the arches of your feet. Squeeze the outside of your shins toward each other.
- Bring the top of your thighs up and back, engaging the quads. Rotate your thighs slightly inward, and widen your sitting bones.
- Tuck in your tailbone slightly without rounding your

lower back. Lift the back of your thighs but release
your buttocks. Keep your hips leveled.

- Bring your pelvis to its neutral position. Do not let
  your front hip bones point down or up; keep pointing
  them forward. Gently bring your belly in slightly.
- As you inhale, lengthen through your torso. As you
  exhale, release your shoulder blades away from your
  head, toward the back of your waist.
- Widen across your collarbones, keeping your
  shoulders in line with the sides of your body.
- Keep your arms straight with fingers extended.
- Lengthen your neck. Your ears, shoulders, hips, and
  ankles are all in one line.
- Keep your breathing smooth and even and with each
  inhale, feel your spine elongating.
- Softly gaze forward toward the horizon line. Hold
  the pose building for up to one minute.

Other yoga poses that could be helpful to fight inflammation
are the Downward Dog, Warrior I, Triangle, Tree, and Child
poses. You will find later on in this book instructions on how
to practice these poses.

PHYSICAL STRATEGIES FOR PAIN MANAGEMENT AND RELIEF

IMPROVE MOBILITY – Changing your body posture may help to reduce pain. Adjusting your body posture can help release pressure over areas where bones are close to the skin surface or reduce areas of swelling; it can give a general feeling of comfort. If you are in pain, you may hesitate to modify your position for fear you will increase pain or damage an area, but avoiding to move because you are afraid of pain can cause several problems. If you are afraid, remember to change your position safely and comfortably. If you cannot move on your own during a yoga session, ask the yoga therapist to help you. Using a yoga prop such as a bolster, cushion, foam block, and/or a belt is helpful.

Exercise is effective in managing pain. Staying a long time without exercise can decrease the body size. This will cause an unwelcome change in the body's structure and metabolism. The heart rate may rise unnecessarily when doing a physical activity, the bones and muscles will waste. With time, inactivity might lead to diminished ability to remain active for a long time, to recover from, and have immunity to trauma, wounds or fatigue.

According to a study by the Mayo Clinic, leading a sedentary lifestyle causes excessive body weight and fat that increase the risk for diabetes, high blood pressure and other health problems.

Physical exercise releases chemicals in our body called endorphins. The release of endorphins in the body due to gentle yoga stretches and movements help promote natural pain reduction and feelings of well-being. A regular and safe yoga practice helps to reduce muscle tension, increase the movement of lymph throughout the body, reduce the risk of blood clots, and support an improved range of motion of the joins. This promotes increased general function.

BEHAVIORAL STRATEGIES FOR PAIN MANAGEMENT AND RELIEF

THE FOLLOWING PHYSICAL, intellectual, and emotional strategies are approaches to help manage pain. Their use can be very effective when done under the direction of a qualified instructor.

Relaxation combines physical and behavioral methods. We can do it with simple, measured breathing techniques and visualization. A simple deep yogic breathing (instructions follow) can change the physical sensation of tension to a feeling of relaxation and can cause a change in body chemistry. Relaxation techniques minimise physical and emotional tension and encourage the release of endorphins.

Guided imagery can be useful in encouraging relaxation and pain relief. The image or visualization must be meaningful to you and must give you comfort. Discuss with your yoga therapist the images that you find helpful in reaching your goal of being distracted from pain.

Meditation is a focused flow of thought that may have a relaxing effect on the meditator. It is a learned skill.

Receiving a systematic instruction from a qualified meditation instructor and a regular practice are required to relieve pain or help forget it.

Mindfulness Meditation is known for reducing inflammation. Researchers associate high levels of inflammation with a less than optimal functioning of the immune system, and to disease. The regular practice of mindfulness meditation improves the functioning of the immune system that in turn enhances the defense against infection and disease. Several studies at the University of California have shown the positive results of the practice of mindfulness meditation leading to a better functioning of the immune system.

BALANCING THE IMMUNE SYSTEM – STRESS MANAGEMENT

THE FOUNDATION of good health is a balanced immune system that functions optimally. Illness and malaise arise when the immune system is imbalanced.

Yoga, when practiced regularly and safely, works to restore balance at all levels – physical, emotional, and mental. The brain, the endocrine, respiratory, nervous and circulatory systems work together to bring the body into balance and restore the immune system to its optimal functioning.

Yoga is an effective tool to manage stress. The immune system must maintain the different aspects of the systems in a state of restful alertness, watching for threatening situations. When the body becomes chronically stressed, the immune system either turns against itself and autoimmune disease(s) arise or becomes so tired that it cannot do its job optimally. That is why reducing stress through the practice of yoga is essential to the health of the immune system.

Increased body awareness – the different systems of the body communicate with each other. By increasing body awareness,

Yoga improves the capability of the immune system to receive and transfer information from and to all areas of the body.

Digestive system—the digestive system functions well in a stress-free environment. Yoga poses and breathing techniques massage and hydrate the digestive areas physically and energetically.

Nervous and endocrine systems – the immune system works with these two to balance the body's metabolism and maintain homeostasis that allows the entire body to function optimally. Homeostasis is the tendency to a relatively stable balance between interdependent elements, especially as maintained by physiological processes. The practice of yoga poses and breathing techniques reduces stress that is important for the nervous system, and massages the glands, which results in optimizing the communication between these systems.

Allergies – allergies are pointless reactions to threats that are perceived as greater than they really are. Yoga practitioners face challenges positively and seek creative solutions. Altruistic and positive states of mind boost the functioning of the immune system.

Body Awareness exercise

- Lie back on a thick blanket or a yoga mat and relax.
- See yourself in a place that makes you feel safe and supported. Take a few minutes to plunge yourself into this feeling of safety.
- Imagine yourself surrounded with a gentle protective light. Pay attention to the color of the light and how it glows strongly in some areas of your body and less strongly in other areas. Notice the sensation of this

light, its color, shape, texture? Describe it to yourself.

- Now, tune into your breath as breath is an essential component to optimal health for the immune system.
- Observe effortlessly the rise and fall of your abdomen in sync with the breath.
- Place one or both hands on your abdomen and when you inhale imagine yourself breathing in the color and a feeling of safety and support. When you exhale, breathe out any feeling of malaise. When you next inhale, draw in more protective energy and when you next exhale, breathe out any feeling of malaise.
- Start with 2 to 5 minutes. With practice, you can increase this exercise to 10 to 15 minutes.

HOW TO MEDITATE AND HOW TO BE MINDFUL

Mindfulness and Mindfulness Meditation

MINDFULNESS IS the awareness of the external life. Meditation is the awareness of the inner life. Mindfulness is being aware of what you are doing when you are doing it. Meditation is the formal practice of finding peace within that is achieved when mental monologue shrinks.

What is Mindfulness?

To be mindful is to listen to your body, listen to your heart, listen to your mind, and live your life with intention. Mindfulness is the way we live every moment of our life when we walk, talk, work, or do any other activity.

Listen to your Body and follow how you feel – Sometimes, we are so taken with daily living that we do not pay attention to our body's clear cues to keep us healthy.

Listen to your Heart – Trust your intuition and follow your joy. Intuition can take many forms and we can sharpen it. Being grateful is powerful and brings healing. Studies show that being grateful has a deep-rooted and long-lasting outcome on our body. Appreciate the here and now. Celebrate life's moments. You are the key to a warm heart, and a healthier happier you. Be kind to yourself. Make and keep a group of supportive people around you as our happiness is in the depth of our relationships.

Listen to your Mind – Keep your brain sharp and happy, read, study, use your imagination, and visualize your day ahead in the morning to help you reach your potential.

What is Mindfulness Meditation?

Mindfulness meditation involves focusing on the breath or bodily sensations without judgement, noticing distracting thoughts as they occur, and returning to the present moment.

Mindfulness is when we are aware of our experiences as they happen. This awareness is the focus of the meditation.

Usually, we are fine in the present moment, but when we are diagnosed with a chronic illness, we might feel afraid, sad and anxious about what will happen. We risk getting stuck in the past and ruminating, or getting anxious about the future.

According to Jon Kabat-Zinn, who founded the mindfulness-based stress reduction program offered by medical centers and hospitals, the practice of mindfulness meditation involves seven main features relating to attitudes. They are non-judging, patience, an open mind, trust, effortless, tolerance, and letting go.

The Health Benefits of Mindfulness Meditation

Many health professionals strongly recommend meditation. Research proves that a regular practice of mindfulness meditation can lessen the symptoms of pain, anxiety, and depression in patients with chronic pain and help manage stress, pain, and illness. Many psychological studies have revealed that regular meditators are happier and enjoy better relationships than those who do not meditate or who meditate occasionally. Studies have shown that meditation strengthens the immune system and is useful against colds, flu, and other diseases.

The mind plays a role in stress and stress-related diseases. Meditation influences a variety of physiological processes of the autonomic system in lowering blood pressure and reducing general excitement and emotional reactions. Practicing mindfulness meditation help to decrease recurring negative thoughts, reduce stress, and improve states of mind. Mindfulness is ideal for an increased awareness of the harmony of mind and body, and how thoughts, feelings, and behaviors can influence emotions and physical and spiritual health.

People who are motivated to improve their health, happiness, and well-being can meditate. You can practice mindfulness every day. You can do any activity mindfully and any activity becomes a practice in mindfulness. This regular practice becomes part of your style of living.

Why do we sometimes find it hard to meditate?

As a yoga and meditation teacher, I have heard many excuses. Some of them are:

I've tried it but I'm not good at this.

Not enough time.

I cannot sit still for too long.

I have too many thoughts.

How to Practice a Basic Mindfulness Meditation

Make sure you will not be interrupted throughout your meditation and switch off all electronic devices.

- Sit comfortably on a cushion or a chair in a way that helps you stay awake. You can lie down if you prefer or walk slowly.
- If you feel alert, close your eyes. If you feel tired, keep your eyes open.
- Begin by taking 2 to 3 deep breaths.
- Let go of thoughts of the past and future and allow your body and mind to relax.
- Breathe normally during the meditation.
- Do not focus on anything specific but be fully aware of what is going on in the present moment.
- If thoughts, sounds, feelings, or physical sensations enter your awareness, gently bring your attention back to your breathing.
- Sit quietly for 10 to 20 minutes while observing your breath.
- If you are in the habit of keeping a journal and writing your thoughts, write how you felt during and after your meditation. Was it hard to meditate? Were you able to bring your attention back to your breathing when you noticed thoughts, sounds, feelings, or physical sensations? Did you feel more relaxed afterward?

BREATHING TECHNIQUES

Diaphragmatic Breathing

THE DIAPHRAGM IS a large muscle shaped like a dome at the base of the lungs. This breathing technique help you use the diaphragm correctly while breathing to strengthen it, decrease the work of breathing by slowing your breathing rate, decrease oxygen demand, and use less effort and energy to breathe.

When you first learn diaphragmatic breathing, it may be easier for you to lie down. As you get used to this practice, you can do it sitting in a chair at which time you will sit comfortably, with your shoulders, head and neck aligned and relaxed.

Start with 5 to 10 minutes of practice up to 3 to 4 times a day. Slowly, increase the practice time. It is better if you breathe only through the nose, and keep your mouth closed.

- Lie on your back on a mat or a thick blanket on the floor or in bed if you need to. If you feel like it, bend your knees and put a pillow under your head to support it. You can also put a pillow under your knees to support your legs.

- Place one hand on your upper chest, and the other hand just below your rib cage to feel your diaphragm move as you breathe.
- Breathe in slowly through your nose so that your stomach moves against your hand. The hand on your upper chest stays still.
- Gently tighten your stomach muscles, letting them fall toward in as you exhale. The hand on your upper chest stays still.

Full Yogic Breathing

Caution:

Your intention is to develop your capacity for moving the breath mindfully and effortlessly.

As you become more comfortable with this practice, you can integrate this style of breathing more in your day-to-day activities.

Benefits:

A calming effect on the mind; accelerates the removal of impurities from the blood, adds more oxygen to the brain, and revitalizes the endocrine system.

How to Practice:

- Sit comfortably or lie down. If you are sitting, make sure that your pelvic bones are rooted into the surface beneath you and your spine is straight. If you prefer to lie down, lie on your back and relax your entire body.

- Gently close your eyes and take a few moments to settle in. Close your mouth and breathe only through the nose. Become aware of your body. Start by observing the natural flow of your breath. Let go of any thoughts and allow yourself to be completely in the present moment.
- Place your right hand on your abdomen and monitor your breathing. Start counting the number of seconds needed for your hand to move up as you inhale and move down as you exhale - this is the natural rhythm of your breath.
- Place the thumbs of both hands under your armpits and spread your fingers wide apart covering a large number of ribs.
- Inhale deep through your nose sending air from your abdomen to your rib cage - notice how your ribs separate and fills up air.
- Exhale through your nose and feel that your abdomen goes down first then your rib cage.
- REPEAT A FEW TIMES.
- Now place your left hand on your collar bone and your right hand on your abdomen.
- Breathe and feel how when you inhale the air fills your lungs like a wave rippling from your abdomen to your rib cage and to your chest.
- Observe this full breathing.
- Now exhale slowly through the nose to the count of 8; watch the air going out.
- Inhale slowly to the count of 8.
- Exhale slowly to the count of 8.

- Keep your attention on the rippling movements of the air.
- Notice the calming effect of this breathing. Frustration and fatigue leave you during the exhalation; peace and detachment come with each inhalation.
- This completes one round of this breathing practice. If your exhalation is followed by a natural pause, take a moment before beginning the next round. Then, draw a fresh inhalation into the lower abdomen.
- After several rounds of this breathing exercise (you can start with 5 minutes and do up to 15 minutes each time), allow your breathing to return to normal for one to two minutes before gently opening your eyes and bringing your practice to a close.
- Then, before you move on to your next activity, pause briefly to notice how you feel. Are you more refreshed, awake, and relaxed? How did your practice affect or benefit you today?

Alternate Nostril Breathing

Caution:

No holding the breath for pregnant women or individuals who suffer from high blood pressure, epilepsy or asthma.

If it is challenging to hold the breath to a certain count, do what you can until you feel comfortable applying the count in the instructions.

Benefits:

Calms the mind, soothes anxiety and stress, balances left and right hemisphere of the brain, and promotes clear thinking.

- Using the right hand, bend the forefinger and middle finger toward the palm of the hand; keep the thumb, ring and pinkie in the air.
- To do one round, close off the right nostril with the thumb and exhale through the left nostril to the count of 8; inhale into the left nostril to the count of 4; close both nostrils (the thumb closes the right nostril and the ring and pinkie fingers close the left nostril) and hold to the count of 16; open the right nostril (the ring and pinkie close the left nostril) and exhale through the right to the count of 8, then inhale into the right nostril, close both nostrils and hold the breath to the count of 16 then open the left and exhale through the left nostril.
- Do 3 rounds.

YOGA PRACTICE

A YOGA POSE or posture (or asana in the Sanskrit language) is a steady and comfortable position. It is mastered by a relaxed effort that helps to reduce the tendency for restlessness.

A complete yoga session is done in a specific order that usually starts with some relaxation and deep yogic breathing (pranayama), warm ups, yoga poses (asanas), yoga pose flows (vinyasa), breathing locks (bandhas), hand gestures (mudras), sometimes contemplation, and finally meditation. The yoga therapist is the one who proposes and recommends the best combination of postures and breathing techniques and the optimal number of poses to practice. The instruction for each pose includes implicit instructions for each of the five koshas. Yoga poses aim to explore and harmonize the whole person.

Yoga practice flows from one pose to another. Every practice builds on the previous one. One step leads to another one. Practicing poses effortlessly and mindfully enhances the beneficial aspects of the practices of the previous poses. This brings about more insight and completion from the current pose you are doing.

Breathing — learning to breathe properly and slowly helps you understand the veiled power of the breath. The breath brings the practice into an interrelated whole.

Warms-ups will teach you to move steadily and rhythmically, in harmony with the breath without forcing toward a goal. This improves blood circulation and the flow of prana in the body which helps the muscles be prepared for change. An increased energy level follows, which strengthens the immune system and helps prepare for the practice itself.

You can better hear the messages of your body with yoga poses as you develop sensitivity and self-restraint. You will then sense the distinction between stretch, strength, strain and pain. You will be able to regulate the pace of your movements, adjust the effort level, and handle pain with awareness. It is common knowledge that a regular and safe yoga practice leads to improvement in balance as shown by several research studies on yoga. The flow of yoga poses strengthens the mind by developing an unbroken awareness of breath. This develops the ability to keep your effort without creating stress. Yoga flows incorporate the yoga motions into daily life activities so you can take the practice with you wherever you go. Your yoga therapist will propose a tailored sequence of yoga poses especially for you.

Bandhas enhance the breathing function. They change breathing into an internal exercise that restores lost energy and boosts energy productivity. They allow the yoga practice to quiet the mind.

Mudras are mostly gestures of the hands, though they may involve the entire body. Their benefits are fully realized when applied to meditation practice.

Practice yoga with pleasure and joy if you want to get the full benefits. If not, you might lose the perseverance to continue.

POPULAR YOGA POSES

ALWAYS REMAIN UNDER THE THRESHOLD OF PAIN. If any part hurts, stop doing the movement. Breathe normally. When you come out of a pose, take a moment to notice its effects.

See Annex 5 to learn about movements you want to avoid if you have an autoimmune condition.

Yoga props – A yoga prop is an object used to help the practice of yoga. Objects like a mat, blanket, bolster, block, belt, and a meditation cushion. Props help yoga practitioners at all levels receive the benefits of a pose over time without exceeding their limit. Props allow you to do poses and breathing exercises with comfort and stability.

Permissions - "The images are Tummee.com copyright and licensed from them. Tummee.com is a yoga sequencing software for yoga teachers."

The yoga poses here appear in an alphabetical order. Send me an email if you want to know how to modify a pose to suit you.

BODY ALIGNMENT

- Sit on a firm cushion or folded blanket. Wiggle to feel that you are sitting evenly on your buttocks. Sit cross-legged with knees as close to the floor as possible, your hips slightly elevated and feeling comfortable.
- If you prefer to sit in a chair, find a posture that gives you stability. Let your spine be as straight as possible without stiffening your upper body. Avoid tilting forward or slouching back.
- Now lift the area between your hips and your waist, then the area between your waist and your shoulders. Lengthen the nape of the neck with chin slightly tucked in.
- Imagine an orange balloon soaring above your head pulling the crown of your head toward the ceiling.
- Hold this pose for 1 to 2 minutes.

BRIDGE POSE (SETUBANHASANA)

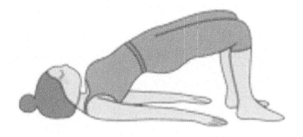

Caution:

To reduce knee pain, place a block between the thighs and press, or under your buttocks or hips for support.

Keep the spine in a straight line from shoulders to knees.

Benefits:

Strengthens the back, buttocks, legs and ankles.

Opens the chest and hips.

Stimulates Samana, Prana and Udana vayus and balances the 3rd, 4th, and 5th chakras.

- Lie on your back with the knees bent, the feet parallel and open at hip-width, and the ankles directly under the knees.
- Inhale, gently arch the low back, keeping the shoulders and the sacrum on the floor.
- Exhale, rest the low back into the floor and tuck the tailbone, engaging the bandhas.
- Inhale and keep the tuck of the pelvis, press the feet into the floor and lift the torso off the floor.
- Exhale as you release the spine into the floor.
- Repeat the cycle 2 to 3 times.

CHAIR POSE (UTKATASANA)

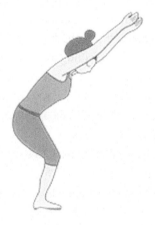

Caution:

If you have knee pain, start with your back against the wall and a block between the thighs; or lie on the floor with your feet against the wall.

Benefits:

Strengthen the supporting muscles of all the major joints.

Develops core strength.

Massages the abdominal organs and improves digestion.

Stimulates Samana, Vyana, Prada, and Apana vayus and balances the 1st, 2nd and 3rd chakras.

- Start in the Mountain pose, aligning the pelvis and the shoulder to be stable. Engage Mulabandha and Uddiyanabandha and lengthen the torso.
- As you inhale, lift the kneecaps and raise the arms to shoulder height in front of the body.
- As you exhale, use the strength of your core to lower the pelvis as if you are sitting in a chair.
- Breathe normally.
- Keep your sacrum lengthening toward the floor and the abdomen drawn back to the spine to reduce curvature in the lower back.
- Bring the rib cage slightly back to keep the torso in alignment with the pelvis.
- Stretch out the fingertips and draw the upper arm bones back into the shoulder joint.
- Keep your shoulders down away from the ears, and direct your gaze gently in a way to keep your neck aligned with your spine.
- Keep the muscles of the legs hugging the bones and engage your legs to protect your knees.
- Find a balance between engagement and easing.
- When you want to come out of the pose, extend your legs and bring your arms by your side coming into the Mountain pose.

CHILD POSE (GARBHASANA)

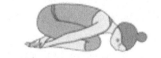

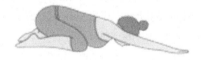

Caution:

Avoid if you suffer from a degenerative disc of the spine.

If pregnant or have a knee, neck or low back pain, use blankets or a rolled-up towel under the ankles, behind the knees, under the hips and/or under the chest and head to feel comfortable.

Benefits:

Facilitates forward flexion in the spine, hips and knees.

Heals, relaxes and rejuvenates the whole body.

Stimulates Samana and Udana vayus and balances all 7 chakras.

- Start on your hand and knees in the Table pose and place the tops of the feet on the floor.
- Rest back on your heels and place your arms by your sides, or stretched in front of you, and rest the forehead on the floor or on a prop.
- Press your pelvis back on their heels and lengthen the spine forward.
- With your shoulders down away from your ears, stretch your hands gently back and turn the palms up. If having your abdomen on your thighs is uncomfortable, open the knees wide.
- Gently engage the bandhas and lengthen the spine from the front and back of the body, creating space in the abdomen and the spine.
- Sense the massage of the organs within the abdominal cavity.
- Soften your spine, and send a feeling of rest and safety to your entire nervous system.
- To come out of this pose, place your hands under the shoulders fingers pointing forward, gently press the hands into the floor and come sitting on your calves and heels.
- Then either sit down or stand up.

COBRA POSE (BHUJANGASANA)

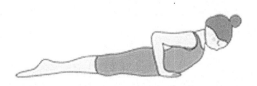

Caution:

Avoid if you have recent or chronic injury to the knees, back, arms or shoulders, pregnancy or recent abdominal surgery.

Benefits:

Opens the chest and strengthens the core body, aligns the spine and invigorates the kidneys and nervous system.

- Lie down on your belly, with the chin on the floor,

palms flat on the floor under the shoulders and legs together.

- Pull up the kneecaps, squeeze the thighs and buttocks, and press the pubic bone down into the floor.
- Without using the arms, inhale and lift the head and chest off the floor, keeping the neck in line with the spine.
- With your elbows close to your sides, press down into your palms and use the arms to lift you up even higher. Drop your shoulders down away from your ears and press the chest back. Remember to keep your legs, buttocks, and pubic bone pressing down into the floor.
- Breathe in and out holding for 3 breaths.
- To release: exhale and slowly lower your chest and head to the floor.

COW'S HEAD POSE (GOMUKHASANA)

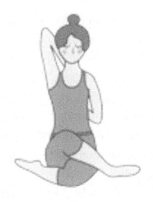

Caution:

Practice correct alignment to help prevent rotator cuff injury.

If you have a knee, hip, or low back pain, place a bolster under your hips, or place a rolled small towel under each ankle.

If you cannot clasp your hands behind your back, use a tie to bring them closer to each other.

Benefits:

Opens the buttocks and deep rotator muscles of the hip; good for sciatica.

Massages the digestive and reproductive organs.

Massages the lymph nodes of the groin and underarms giving immune support.

Stimulates Samana and Prana vayus and activates the lower 4 chakras.

- Come on your hands and knees into the Table pose. Cross the left knee in front of the right, placing the right knee against the back of the left knee.
- Open your feet apart and press the tops of the feet on the floor.
- Press the thighs together to get support and place your buttocks back on the floor or on a prop. Both sitting bones must rest on whatever you are sitting on so that the pelvis is level.
- Engage Mulabandha and Uddiyanabandha and lift the rib cage up out of the pelvis.
- Relax your shoulders and bring the shoulder blades down your back.
- Stretch the right arm up overhead and bend it at the elbow so that the fingers rest right behind the right shoulder. Draw the breastbone back and in to avoid arching the back.
- Bring your left arm behind your back and reach up to

clasp the fingers of the right hand. If necessary, use a strap or a tie to bring your hands closer.

- Once the hands are joined or as close as can be, bring the elbows gently away from each other and create space between the shoulder blades.
- Your torso and gaze are facing forward, and your chin is parallel to the floor.
- As you inhale, engage the bandhas and draw the breath deep into the abdomen.
- As you exhale, allow the energy to rise into the heart to nourish the Heart center.
- Hold the pose for 2 to 3 breaths.
- Release slowly and repeat to the other side.

CROCODILE POSE (MAKARASANA)

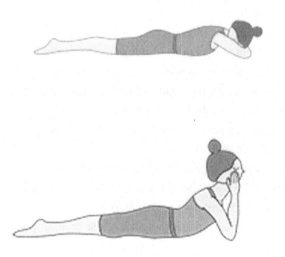

Caution:

Pregnant women should avoid this pose.

If you have neck pain, use a prop to support your forehead, or place 2 bolsters lengthwise end-to-end under your body and support the forehead on the hands to keep the cervical spine neutral.

Benefits:

Lengthens the spine.

Massages the abdominal organs and reproductive system.

Rests the nerves.

Stimulates Samana vayu and balances the 2nd chakra.

- Lie on your belly with elbows bent out to the side, hands on top of each other, and one cheek resting on the hands.
- Rest in this position for several breaths, then turn your head to the opposite side and change the position of your hands.
- Now, bring the forehead to the floor and stretch the arms forward. Walk your fingertips forward, stretching your arms while your legs and back stretch through the legs and feet.
- Keeping this length, bring the arms and legs back in line with your body and bend the elbows and place them directly under the shoulders.
- Place the hands under the jaw and use them to gently bring your head forward lengthening the neck.
- Stay in this pose for a few breaths.
- To come out of the pose, place your hands under the shoulders fingers pointing forward, gently press the hands into the floor and come sitting on your calves and heels.

DOWNWARD DOG POSE (ADHO MUKHA SVANASANA)

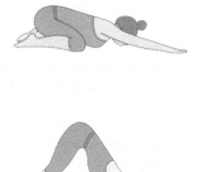

Caution:

If you have wrist or shoulder pain, face a wall, bend at the hips and press the hands into the wall.

To develop strength and alignment in your legs, put a block between the thighs.

Benefits:

Creates integration and balance between upper and lower body.

Strengthen and stretches legs and shoulders.

Calms the nervous system.

Stimulates Prana, Apana and Udana vayus and balances all 7 chakras.

- Come into the child pose, lengthening the arms as you stretch the fingertips forward and bring the upper arm bones back into the shoulder joint.
- Lengthen the spine.
- As you inhale into the Table pose, widen the base of support in the hands by spreading the fingers and pressing into the web between the thumb and index fingers.
- Bring the upper arm bones deeper into the shoulder sockets, and spread the shoulders apart as you press the lower arms toward each other.
- As you exhale, curl the toes under and lift your sitting bones into the air, keeping the knees bent and the heels off the floor.
- Lengthen the arms and spine, to have a straight line of energy from the wrists to the pelvis. Keep the shoulders relaxed and the shoulder blades moving toward the pelvis.
- Engage the bandhas and lift the hips higher into the air as the legs straighten.

- Stretch through the legs and walk the heels from side-to-side to deepen the stretch and, when comfortable, draw both heels toward the floor and hold the pose.
- Find a balance point between the front and the back body, supported in the center by the bandhas, and stay in this position for a few breaths.
- To come out, drop the knees down to the floor and come sitting on your calves and heels.

GODDESS POSE (DEVIASANA OR UTKATA KONASANA)

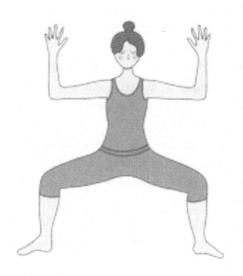

Caution:

Avoid if you have an inguinal hernia.

For knee and ankle pain, you can place your hands on your

thighs for support, or stand with your back against the wall, or lie on the floor with the soles of your feet pressing against the wall.

Benefits:

Strengthens the muscles supporting the joints in the extremities, especially knees and ankles.

Improves circulation to the abdominal organs and legs.

Increases Apana, Vyana and Samana vayus and activates the lower 3 chakras.

- Stand into a wide position with your legs and feet turned out at a 45-degree angle and the arms open at the level of your shoulders.
- Press your feet evenly into the floor.
- Activate Mulabandha by gently drawing the pelvic floor up and activate Uddiyanabandha by drawing the lower abdomen back toward the spine so you can have a stable core.
- As you exhale, bend the knees and let your pelvis move down without arching the low back so that your torso moves down in as much a straight line as possible.
- Bend your knees so that they are over the ankles, your pelvis is not tilting forward or back. Gently let the thighs open as your body moves down.
- Bend the elbows at a 90-degree angle and direct your forearms and hands up, keeping the fingers together and the palms facing forward.
- Lift the rib cage and create space in the chest and back without pressing the shoulder blades together.
- Your chin is parallel to the floor, your eyes gaze

softly to the horizon as you lengthen from the crown of the head.

- The center of the pose is just below the navel. Let the energy radiate from this point to your arms and legs.
- To come out of the pose, lower the arms, and extend the legs then bring them together.

HALF CIRCLE POSE (ARDHA MANDALASANA)

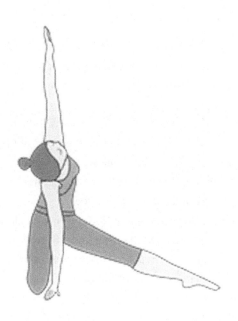

Caution:

Avoid if you have knee pain or injury.

If you have trouble with your wrist, put a foam block under the weight-bearing hand. Modify the pose by having the top arm in line with the body instead of overhead.

Benefits:

Stimulates the entire immune system.

Opens the physical and energetic heart.

Stimulates Vyana, Samana and Udana vayus and balances the 4th chakra.

- Come on your knees. Engage Mulabandha and Uddiyanabandha and lengthen through the crown of the head while pressing down your knees and the tops of your feet.
- Stretch the left leg to the left in line with the torso, and place the sole of the foot on the floor and let the arch of the left foot be in line with the right knee.
- Your right thigh is at a 90-degree angle pressing into the floor from the knees to the toes.
- Place the right hand on the floor or on a block in line with the left arch and the right knee. Spread the fingers wide to form a strong base of support pointing them in the direction of your head.
- Bring your shoulders down away from the ears and lengthen both sides of the rib cage as you lengthen the torso out of the hips.
- Extend the left arm up and overhead and feel energy from the arm up to the fingertips of the extended hand.

- Hold the pose for several breaths making sure that your pelvis and the shoulder girdles (the clavicle and scapula that connect to the arm on each side) are in a neutral position.
- Release the pose, come back to the center on your knees and repeat to the other side.

HALF LOCUST WITH HEAD AND CHEST RAISED POSE (ARDHA SHALABHASANA)

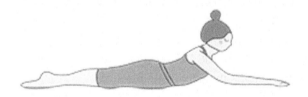

Caution:

Avoid if you have recent or chronic injury to the back or legs, pregnancy or recent abdominal surgery.

Benefits:

Strongly strengthens the core body and the low back muscles, and stimulates the endocrine, nervous and reproductive systems.

- Lie on your belly with the chin on the floor, legs together and your arms next to your body.

- Engage Mulabandha and Uddiyanabandha and as you inhale lift your head and look forward, bring the left arm forward, and point the toes of the right foot, extend the knee and lift the right thigh as high as possible, without strongly pressing the opposite thigh against the floor.
- Breathe normally and hold for 3 breaths.
- To release, exhale and slowly lower the left arm and right thigh to the floor bringing your forehead to the floor.
- Next, inhale and lift your head, stretch the right arm forward, point the toes of the left foot, extend the knee and lift the left thigh as high as possible, without strongly pressing the opposite thigh against the floor.
- Breathe and hold for 3 breaths
- To release, exhale and slowly lower the head, right arm and left thigh to the floor.

HALF WIND RELIEVING POSE
(ARDHA PAVANA MUKTASANA)

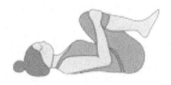

Caution:

Avoid this pose if you have had recent abdominal surgery, hernia, spinal injury or sciatica.

Avoid if you have severe migraine, a slipped disc, advanced stages of spondylitis, or problems with the lower abdomen.

Those with asthma must learn the flow of breath before they practice this pose as pressure around the chest and lungs may cause stress during breathing.

Avoid during menstruation.

Benefits:

Improves digestion and elimination. Help to release unwanted gas/wind.

Gently stretches and heals low back pain.

Relieves tired legs and strengthens the back.

- Lying on your back, tuck the chin into the chest with the head on the floor.
- Gently pull one knee into the chest using the arms, avoiding the ribcage. Interlace the fingers 1 or 2 inches below the kneecap.
- Press the shoulders and the back of the neck down into the floor, keep the elbows close to the sides of the body. Relax the legs, feet and hips.
- Breathe and hold for 3 breaths.
- Exhale and release the arms and the leg to the floor.
- Repeat on the other side.

KNEE TO CHEST POSE (APANASANA)

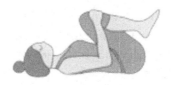

Caution:

Avoid if you suffer from a degenerative disc of the spine.

If you have knee pain, clasp your hands under your knee, or bring one knee to the chest but keep the opposite leg bent with the sole of the foot on the floor.

Benefits:

Massages abdominal organs.

Good for elimination problems such as constipation and menstrual cramps.

Helpful for low back pain.

Stimulates Apana and Samana vayus and balances the lower 2 chakras.

- Lie down on the floor, engage your bandhas, and let your shoulder and pelvis be in a neutral position. Your arms are by your side with the palms turned up.
- Bend the right knee and bring it close to the chest avoiding the ribcage. Interlace the fingers on the shin bone just below the knee.
- Press through the left heel while you bring the right thigh to your body, keeping the pelvis neutral.
- Keep the shoulders down away from the ears.
- Press your leg out through the left heel and draw the head of the left upper leg bone back into the hip joint.
- The low back and pelvis keep in contact with the floor.
- As you exhale, draw the thigh into the abdomen. As you inhale, let the abdomen expand, pushing the shin gently out against the interlaced fingers.
- Notice the rise and fall of the abdomen.
- Rest into the pose with your eyes closed.
- Slowly release the pose and repeat with the other leg.

MOUNTAIN POSE OR STANDING WELL (TADASANA)

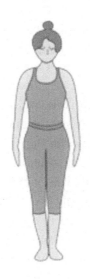

Caution:

If you have leg, hip, spinal or shoulder pain, hyper lordosis or kyphosis, begin with modified poses using the wall or the floor for support.

Benefits:

Good basic alignment for poses.

Supports health in the joints.

Creates space in the abdominal cavity for digestive health.

Stimulates Prana and Apana vayus and balances the 1st chakra.

- Stand with your feet together and your arms at your sides. Gently press your weight evenly on the floor. Breathe steadily and rhythmically. Direct your attention inward and focus on the present moment, letting go of worries and concerns.
- Press lightly your big toes together (separate your heels if you need to). Lift your toes and spread them apart. Then, place them back down on the mat.
- If you have trouble balancing, stand with your feet six inches apart (about 15 cm) or wider, or place a hand on a wall or a chair for support.
- Ground your feet firmly into the earth. Then, lift your ankles and the arches of your feet. Squeeze the outside of your shins toward each other.
- Bring the top of your thighs up and back, engaging the quads. Rotate your thighs slightly inward, and widen your sitting bones.
- Tuck in your tailbone slightly without rounding your lower back. Lift the back of your thighs but release your buttocks. Keep your hips levelled.
- Bring your pelvis to its neutral position. Do not let

your front hip bones point down or up; keep pointing them forward. Gently bring your belly in slightly.

- As you inhale, lengthen through your torso. As you exhale, release your shoulder blades away from your head, toward the back of your waist.
- Widen across your collarbones, keeping your shoulders in line with the sides of your body.
- Keep your arms straight with fingers extended.
- Lengthen your neck. Your ears, shoulders, hips, and ankles are all in one line.
- Keep your breathing smooth and even and with each inhale, feel your spine elongating.
- Softly gaze forward toward the horizon line. Hold the pose building for up to one minute.

PELVIC TILT

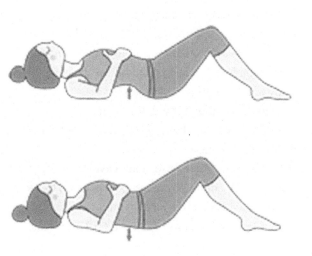

Caution:

Avoid pushing out your abdominal muscles or raising your low back off the floor.

Gently pull your abdominals in to the floor. Imagine pushing your belly button in to your back.

Benefits:

Helps to strengthen the abdominal muscles.

When you relax, strengthen and elongate your muscles, you will help ease back pain.

- Lie on your back, lower the chin slightly down to elongate the nape of the neck and align it with the spine.
- Bend your knees keeping the feet flat on the floor.
- Tuck the buttocks and raise the public bone up. Feel the contact of your waist with the floor.
- Contract the abdomen and lift the insides up toward the chest cavity, creating a hollow under the rib cage.
- Keep on breathing and gently press the navel down toward the spine
- Hold the position for a few seconds.
- Relax, straighten the legs and take a few breaths.
- Repeat once more.
- To come out of the pose, and to avoid hurting your back when coming from a supine position to a sitting one, place your hands under your knees, straighten your legs high and roll back and forth until you gently sit up.

PLANK POSE (CHATURANGA DANDASANA)

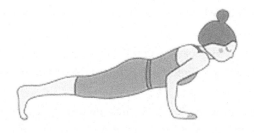

Caution:

If your arms feel weak, keep one knee on the floor or bend your arms. You can also place a foam block under the pubic bone.

Benefits:

Postural stability for the whole body.

Strengthens and aligns the shoulder joints.

Develops the overall fitness level, including heart and lungs.

Stimulates Samana, Vyana, Prana, and Apana vayus and activates the lower three chakras.

- Start in the Table pose and align your body to create stability in the shoulder and pelvis.
- Have your shoulders in a neutral position by relaxing them away from the ears, broadening the upper back, spreading the shoulder blades apart as you widen the front of the chest.
- Spread the fingers wide, with a firm base of support for the hands, pressing down into the pads below the knuckles and into the webs between the thumb and index fingers.
- Keep your head in line with the spine, let your gaze be soft looking down.
- Engage Mulabandha and Uddiyanabandha to support a neutral position of the pelvis and lengthen your spine.
- Stretch the left leg back, tuck the toes under, and lengthen from the heels to the crown of the head. Now stretch the right leg back and come into the plank pose.
- Press the heels back and the crown forward and keep your shoulders away from your ears.
- To be stable in this pose, press the forearms gently toward each other and the upper arms and shoulders moderately away from each other.
- If you feel any shaking or trembling, you can either witness it or simply come out of the pose by dropping one knee at a time to the floor.
- This pose is usually followed by the child pose.

RECLINING BUTTERFLY POSE
(SUPTA BADDHA KONASANA)

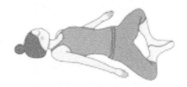

Caution:

Avoid if you have a hip injury.

If pregnant, avoid lying on your back for too long. Have your back supported against a wall or a pile of cushions.

If your hips are tight, place a cushion under each knee or thigh for support.

Benefits:

Externally rotates the hips and improve their mobility.

Help ease upper and lower back pain.

Relieves stress.

Stimulates Apana and Vyana vayus and calms the 1st chakra.

- Sit on the floor and extend your legs. Bring the soles of the feet together and let the knees drop out to the side.
- Lie back either on a mat or a blanket, a bolster, or propped on your forearms. If supported, place your hands on your belly or out to the sides.
- Stay for 5-10 breaths.
- To come out, extend your legs, roll to your side and push your hand on the floor to sit up.

RELIEVE STRESS WITH LEGS-UP-THE-WALL POSE (VIPARITA KARANI)

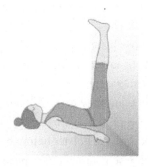

Viparita Karani is usually done near the end of a practice just before the final deep relaxation. Some people start with this pose as it helps them fight fatigue and prepare to do yoga.

Caution:

Avoid if you have glaucoma, high blood pressure, heart disease, acid reflux or hernia, and during menstruation.

Avoid if you have neck and shoulder pain or low back injury.

Benefits:

Calms the mind and eases headaches.

Boosts energy.

Relieves lower-back pain.

- The supported version with a prop may be more relaxing for some people. Whether doing a supported or unsupported version you need a wall or a secure door to rest your legs.
- If you are practicing the supported version, set a bolster or a firm, long pillow on the floor against the wall.
- Begin the pose by sitting with your left side against the wall. Your lower back should rest against the bolster, if using one.
- Gently turn your body to the left and bring your legs up onto the wall. If you are using a bolster, shift your lower back onto the bolster before bringing your legs up the wall. Use your hands for balance as you shift your weight.
- Lower your back to the floor and lie down. Rest your shoulders and head on the floor.
- Shift your weight from side-to-side and bring your buttocks close to the wall. Your arms are at your sides with the palms facing up. If you're using a bolster, have your lower back fully supported by it.
- Let the heads of your thigh bones (the part of the bone that connects in the hip socket) release and relax, dropping toward the back of your pelvis.

- Close your eyes. Hold for 5-10 minutes, breathing with awareness.
- To release, slowly push yourself away from the wall and slide your legs down to the right side. Use your hands to help press yourself back up into a seated position.

RUNNER POSE (ASHWA SANCHALASANA)

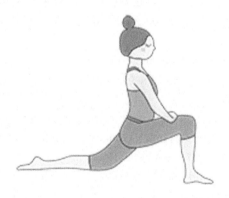

Caution:

Avoid or modify this pose if you have a knee, hip or low back pain, to be comfortable.

Place each hand on a block to relieve tightness in the hip and align the spine with the back leg.

Bend the back knee on the floor at a 90-degree angle and put your hands on the front knee.

Benefits:

Strengthens and aligns the legs.

Opens the hip joints.

Helpful for sciatica.

Massages the digestive and reproductive organs.

Stimulates Samana, Prana and Apana vayus and balances the lower two chakras.

- Start in the Table pose, and engage Mulabandha and Uddiyanabandha to keep the hips and shoulders in a neutral position.
- Lift the right hand and bring the right leg forward, placing the sole of the foot on the floor between the hands.
- Place the right knee right over the right ankle and hug the muscles into the bones to support the knee. Press the right foot in the floor.
- Slide the left knee back so that the left leg is straightened back; keep the left knee on the floor.
- Make sure your pelvis is square by pulling the left side of the pelvis up and the right side back and down.
- Stretch the body in different directions by pressing the front shin forward and the back heel back.
- Release the pose by bringing the back knee down and coming back into the table pose.
- Repeat on the other side.

SEATED FORWARD BEND
(PASCHIMOTTANASANA)

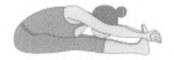

Caution:

Pregnant women should avoid this pose.

Bend the knees if your muscles feel tight.

Hold a strap or a tie around the balls of the feet and keep your spine straight.

Benefits:

Elongates the spine and opens the muscles of the back.

Revitalizes Samana, Prana and Apana vayus, and balances the lower 3 chakras.

- Stand in the Staff pose and press your hands gently on the floor.
- Draw your kneecaps up to engage your thighs while you elongate the legs by pressing out the heels.
- Bend forward from the hip but keep your spine neutral, and slide your hands on your legs as far as comfortable for you.
- Keep your shoulders away from your ears. Elongate your neck to align head with spine.
- As you inhale, lengthen the trunk of your body, and as you exhale, let it come further down toward the top of your thighs but keeping your spine neutral.
- Hold effortlessly for a few breaths letting the breath bring cooling energy to your entire body but especially your abdominal organs.
- To come out of the pose, gently roll back to the Staff pose.

STAFF POSE OR SITTING WELL
(DANDASANA)

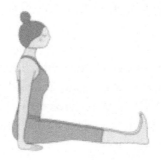

Caution:

If you have low back pain or tight hamstrings, do the pose lying on your back with the arms by your sides.

If you have difficulty sitting upright, sit on a cushion or a foam wedge.

Benefits:

Strengthens the hip flexors.

Strengthens the abdominal area and low back, and stretches the shoulders and the chest.

Creates space for full breathing.

Revitalizes Prana, Samana, Apana, and Vyana vayus, and balances the lower 3 chakras.

- Sit down and stretch your legs in front of you. Place your hands close to your body with the palms pressing into the floor.
- Draw the kneecaps up and lengthen the legs by pressing out through the heels as you ground your sitting bones.
- Engage Mulabandha and Uddiyanabandha and lengthen your torso out of the hips, lifting up.
- Let your muscles and the engaged bandhas support your upper body at a 90-degree angle.
- As you inhale, draw your breath up through the sole of the feet into your core.
- As you exhale allow the breath and the energy to rise up into the torso, lifting the rib cage, lengthening to the crown of the head and sending energy all the way to the fingertips.
- Hold this pose for 3 to 5 breaths and then release.

SUNBIRD POSE (CHAKRAVAKASANA)

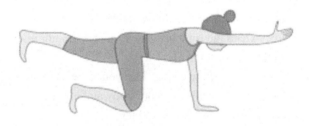

Caution:

If you have back, neck, shoulder, wrist, elbow, knee or shoulder pain, keep both hands on the floor.

If you feel a lack of stability, do it with the side of the body against a wall.

Benefits:

Stabilizes the spine and pelvis.

Good for low back pain.

Activates Mulabandha and Uddiyanabandha fully.

Revitalizes Prana, Apana, Samana, and Vyana vayus, and balances the lower 2 chakras.

- From the Table pose, make sure you are aligned to stabilize the shoulders and pelvis.
- As you inhale, extend the left leg back in a straight line with the spine to have a line of energy from the hip to the crown of the head.
- Keep your bandhas gently engaged, and sense that the pelvis and shoulders are stable when the legs separate.
- Hold this position with the left leg out, the pelvis in a neutral position and the body stable. When you're ready, extend the right arm forward in a straight line with the rest of the body.
- As you inhale, draw energy into your core. As you exhale, radiate it all over your body and use it to support the extended arm and leg.
- Let the energy of your core support you.
- Release the extended arm and leg and come into the Table pose.
- Now repeat to the other side.

SUN SALUTATION (SURYA NAMASKARA)

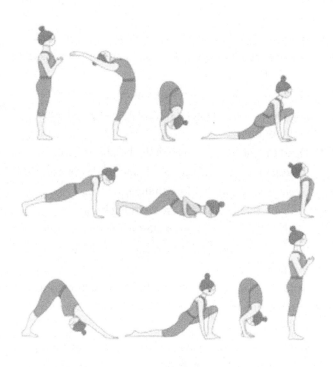

Caution:

Avoid if you have a recent or chronic injury to the knees, hips, or back.

Benefits:

Builds strength and increases flexibility.

If one day you think you have no time for yoga, do at least 1 or 2 rounds of the Sun Salutation.

The Sun Salutation is a series of postures performed in a single, graceful flow. Coordinate each movement with the breath.

1. Begin by standing in Mountain pose with your feet open hip-width apart and hands in prayer pose. Take several breaths.
2. Hands up – On your next inhalation, tilt your pelvis and in one movement raise your arms up and gently arch your back.
3. Head to Knees – As you exhale, bend forward, bending the knees if necessary, and place your hands by your feet, fingers close to the little toes.
4. Lunge – Inhale and step the right leg back.
5. Plank – Exhale and step the left leg back coming into the plank position and hold a little breathing normally.
6. Stick – Lower your knees to the floor, buttocks close to heels, lower your chest to the floor and scroll forward.
7. Cobra – Inhale and stretch forward and up, bending at the waist. Use your arms to lift your torso, bend back as long as it's comfortable and safe. Look

straight ahead. You can keep your arms bent at the elbow.

8. Downward Dog – Exhale, lift from the hips and push the hips up and back.
9. Lunge – Inhale and step the right forward.
10. Head to Knees – Exhale bring the left foot forward and come into head-to-knee position; bend your knees if necessary.
11. Hands-up – Inhale and come up raise slowly while keeping your arms extended.
12. Mountain – Exhale and lower your arms to the sides and bring your hands into a prayer position.
13. Repeat the sequence, stepping with the left leg this time.

SAVASANA – RELAXATION POSE (DONE AT THE END OF THE YOGA PRACTICE)

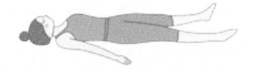

Caution:

Begin with short periods of practice (or none) if you feel depressed or lethargic.

Place props under the head, neck, arms and knees as needed.

Benefits:

Regulates high blood pressure.

Calms and balances the circulatory, digestive, endocrine, lymphatic and immune systems.

Stimulates all 5 vayus and balances all 7 chakras.

- Lie down on your back, let the arms and legs drop open, with the arms about 45-degrees from the side of your body. Make sure you are warm and comfortable and place blankets under or over your body if you must.
- Imagine that you have bitten into a very sour lemon. Feel how your face squint and frown. Clench your teeth and fists, and tighten your buttocks and legs. Hold that tightness for a few seconds and then let it all relax. Notice the immediate change in your body.
- Separate your arms and legs apart.
- Open your eyes - roll them back and close - wait until they become still.
- Separate your teeth and let your lower jaw sag and relax.
- Notice your tongue, feel how limp it is. Let your facial muscles be as limp.
- Turn the head slowly from side to side, bring it back to the center and feel how the neck has loosened.
- Let the whole body sink passively into the floor.
- Feel how limp the arms are, let them hang loosely.
- Become aware of your legs, notice how the thighs and calves have softened, how the ankles have passively flopped sideways.
- Give your tired muscles permission to let go – notice how readily they do it.
- Notice your breathing and how subtle it has become.
- As you inhale, mentally repeat to yourself "I AM", and as you exhale mentally repeat to yourself "RELAXED". Let your mind drift away and imagine your mind as a cloud, slowly dissolving into the

immense blue sky. Enjoy that sense of blissful calm. Keep inhaling "I AM" and exhaling "RELAXED".

Coming out of deep relaxation

- It is important not to open the eyes quickly and jump out of relaxation – you may have reached a much deeper state than you appreciate – so a steady return to daily awareness is essential.
- Keep your eyes closed.
- Wiggle your toes, circle your ankles, and stretch your legs.
- Rotate both wrists.
- Stretch the arms, roll the shoulders, yawn lazily, stretch the whole body and feel that you are awakening from a pleasant refreshing dream.
- Sit up slowly and straighten your back. Your eyes are still closed.
- Mentally re-align the body, the mind, and the emotions.
- Compare how you feel now with the way you felt at the beginning of the session, notice the improvement.
- Open your eyes and stretch again pleasurably.
- Stand up and stretch more, really enjoying a sense of looseness and aliveness.
- You can repeat whenever you feel stressed or cannot fall asleep.

SPHINX POSE (SALAMBA BHUJANGASANA)

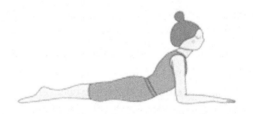

Caution:

Avoid if you are pregnant.

If you have low back pain, do all back bending poses carefully or place a bolster under the chest for support.

Benefits:

Correct alignment of shoulders.

Gentle elongation of the spine.

Stimulates Samana and Prana vayus, and balances the 2nd and 4th chakras.

- Lie down in crocodile pose with the body elongated on the floor and arms stretched.
- Bend your elbows and bring them back to rest under the shoulders, with the upper arms perpendicular to the floor.
- Place the forearms parallel to each other and actively press them into the floor.
- Spread the fingers wide apart with the middle fingers facing forward. Press into the base of support between the thumb and index fingers and under the pads of the knuckles.
- Have your shoulders down away from the ears and slide the shoulder blades down your back.
- Bring the breastbone forward and elongate back with the legs.
- Keep the low back neutral and the buttocks soft.
- Let the breath move gently up and down the spine. As you inhale, elongate the space between the vertebrae, and as you exhale relax the spine.
- Rest in this pose and allow the energy of the heart to expand.

STANDING TWIST POSE

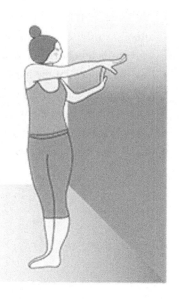

Caution:

This is a warm-up pose to prepare the body for more intense yoga poses/yoga flow.

Those who do not have the strength, flexibility or stability to do a standing twist use the wall as a prop.

Benefits:

Benefits a good number of muscles including arms, shoulders, back, neck and the psoas.

Activates the 5th chakra.

- Stand with the side of your body about 30 cm away from the wall, your feet are parallel and open at hip-width.
- With your pelvis motionless, rotate the front of the torso toward the wall and place both hands on the wall at the level of your shoulders.
- Use the support of the hands to gently rotate the torso to the wall as the pelvis makes a counter rotation away from the wall.
- Look over the shoulder and breathe normally.
- Come back to the center and repeat the other side.

SEATED SPINAL TWIST POSE
(ARDHA MATSYENDRASANA)

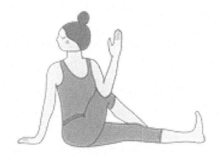

Caution:

Approach with caution if you have abdominal pain, recent surgery or back pain.

Benefits:

Twisting Poses help restore the natural range of motion of your spine, cleanse your organs, and stimulate circulation.

Relaxes and releases mental tensions bringing you in the present moment.

Stimulates Samana vayu and balances the 2nd and 3rd chakras.

- Sit down and extend your legs. Bend the right leg and cross it over the left extended leg.
- Bring the top of the thighs into the floor and lift from the pelvis. Lift the crown of the head and draw your shoulders down.
- Place the left hand outside the right knee and the right hand behind your back as close to the sacrum as comfortable. Point your fingers back.
- As you inhale, lengthen the spine and lift the rib cage.
- As you exhale, deepen the twist.
- Keep the bandhas engaged to firm the abdomen and the low back.
- Release, come back to the center and repeat to the other side.

SUPINE CRESCENT MOON POSE (BANANASANA)

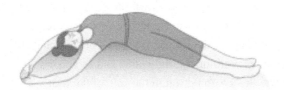

Caution:

Opens the ribs and intercostal muscles allowing fuller breathing.

If you have heart disease, high blood pressure, stroke, spinal injuries or low back pain, do this pose with your arms at your side.

Benefits:

Massages abdominal organs.

Deeply relaxes the nervous system.

Stimulates Prana, Apana and Samana vayus, and balances the 3rd chakra.

- Lie down on your back with the arms resting by your side. Stretch from the heels to the crown of the head and engage the bandhas to bring the pelvis in a neutral position.
- Bring the right arm overhead, lengthening the fingertips away from the body as you gently pull the upper arm into the shoulder joint
- Walk the heels to the left and walk the upper body to the left so that your entire body forms a long crescent moon from the outer heel of the right foot to the right fingertips.
- Imagine a line of energy down the center of the body dividing the body from right to left. Notice the opening side of the Crescent Moon. As you inhale draw the breath up the right side, and as you exhale release the tension through the sole of the foot.
- Release slowly back to the center and repeat to the other side.

STANDING FORWARD BEND
(UTTANASANA)

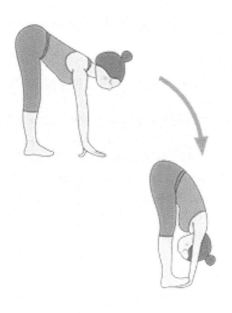

Caution:

Avoid if you suffer from a degenerative disc of the spine.

Caution should be used for pregnancy, recent abdominal surgery, high blood pressure, and sinus or eye problem; recent or chronic injury to the legs, hips, back or shoulders.

If you cannot easily touch the floor with your knees straight, place each hand on a yoga block placed at the outer edge of each foot.

Benefits:

Lengthens the spinal column and stretches the backs of the legs and the back muscles; stimulates digestive, nervous and endocrine systems.

Works on Udana, Samana, and Prana vayus, and balances all the chakras.

- From a standing position, bring the feet hip width apart, parallel.
- Lift up the toes, spread them wide and place them back on the floor. Feel your weight evenly distributed on your feet, not leaning forward or back.
- Pull up the kneecaps, squeeze the thighs and tuck the tailbone under. The legs are straight without locking the knees back.
- As you exhale, hinge forward at the hips. Bend the knees enough to bring the palms flat to the floor and the head close to the knees.
- Feel the spine stretching in opposite directions as you pull the head down and in and press the hips up.
- Breathe and hold for 3 breaths, actively pressing the belly into the thighs on the inhalation.

- To come out of the pose, bend the knees keeping the back straight, inhale the arms out to the sides, and then bring your arms and torso up back into mountain pose.

TABLE/CAT POSE (MARJARIASANA)

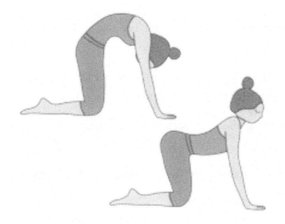

Caution:

If you have knee or wrist pain, use a foam wedge under the heels of the hands or the knees.

If you have neck injuries, keep the head in line with the torso, not dropping it forward or back.

Pregnant women and those with back injuries should only perform Cow Pose, by bringing the spine back to neutral between poses — do not let the belly drop between repetitions.

If you have back pain, lie on your back with your feet up against the wall.

Benefits:

Stretches the back torso and neck.

Softly stimulates and strengthens the abdominal organs.

Opens the chest, encouraging the breath to become slow and deep.

Coordinating movement with breathing relieves stress and calms the mind.

Brings the spine into correct alignment and can help prevent back pain when practiced regularly.

Strengthens the low back and abdomen with a lengthened spine.

Generates stability in wrists, elbows, shoulders, hips and knees.

Facilitates Prana and Apana vayus, and activates the lower 2 chakras.

- Come on your hands and knees with the knees directly under the hips and the wrists directly under the shoulders.
- Spread the fingers wide apart and press the web between thumb and index fingers firmly into the floor.

- Press the tops of the feet into the floor to form a firm support for your back.
- Lengthen from your tailbone to the crown of the head, relax the shoulders away from the ears, and take your shoulder down away from your ears.
- Widen across the upper back and the front of the chest. Avoid hyperextending your elbows.
- As you exhale, round your back up starting the movement at the tailbone. Let the crown of the head fold down naturally and let your chin come close to the chest. When you reach full exhalation, draw the abdomen in toward the spine.
- As you inhale, and starting at the tailbone, let the spine come down toward the floor, open the chest open and lift your head and look forward or look up.
- Continue this movement slowly and gently, for several breaths, noticing the moment when the spine get to the neutral position.

TREE POSE (VRKASANA)

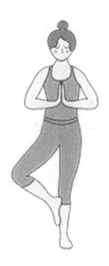

Caution:

If you have leg pain or weakness, lie on the floor and press the foot into a wall.

If you lack balance, use the wall or the back of a chair for support.

Benefits:

Strengthens and stabilizes the legs.

Helpful for knee pain.

Improves balance.

Work on Samana, Prana, Apana and Vyana vayus, and balances the lower 3 and the 6th chakras.

- Begin in Mountain pose. Bend the right knee and bring the sole of the right foot to the inner calf or the inner left thigh with the heel against the calf or the thigh.
- Press the sole of the foot and the inner side against each other.
- Drop the right hip down to lengthen the right waist and press the right knee out and down away from the center of the body to be at the same level as the pelvis.
- Press the right leg back and have the pelvis facing forward.
- Bring the arms slowly out to the side at the level of shoulder and then into a prayer pose.
- Draw the lower ribs back and down to lengthen the low back and to align the rib cage with the pelvis.
- Elongate the crown of the head and look at the horizon. Relax your eyes, jaw, and forehead.
- After a few breaths, come back to the center and do the same on the other side.

TRIANGLE POSE (TRIKONASANA)

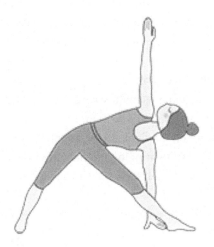

Caution:

If you have sacroiliac, low back or hip pain, keep the front knee slightly bent and place the front hand just above or below the knee.

Keep your gaze forward if you have neck pain.

Benefits:

Aligns the legs, hips and arms.

Creates a gentle rotation of the spine from a lengthened position.

Helps create fuller breathing.

Balances the entire being physically and energetically.

Balances Vyana and Udana vayus, and activates all chakras especially the heart chakra.

- Stand with legs wide open.
- Turn the right foot out at a 90-degree angle and the left foot back at a 45-degree angle, with the front heel in line with the arch of the back heel.
- Press both feet into the floor, activate the legs and pull up the knee caps.
- Lift the arms up to shoulder height and stretch the fingertips in different direction.
- Reach through the right arm and stretch to the right as far as possible bringing the right hip joint back and down as the left hip move up and a little forward.
- Lower both sides of the torso evenly to the right, and place the right hand on the right shin for support.
- Gently draw the pelvic floor and the lower abdomen in, so that the pubic bone moves up toward the navel and the sacrum slides downward, reducing excessive lumbar curve and lengthening the spine from the sacrum to the crown of the head.
- Rotate the chest open, stretching the left arm up.

- Draw your neck back as the shoulder blades slide down your back.
- Tuck the chin and either look in front of you or rotate the head up, keeping your neck in line with the spine.
- Open across the front of the hips, keeping the back hip forward just enough to keep the sides of the torso of even length, with the spine in a neutral, lengthened position.
- Release the pose and come up.
- Take a few moments to absorb the benefit of this pose, then repeat to the other side.

WARRIOR POSE I
(VIRABHADRASANA I)

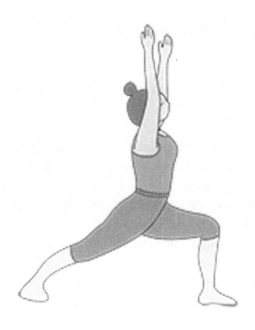

Caution:

Injury to the knees or the hips can make this pose difficult. If you have weak knees or pain, press the front knee into a folded blanket on the seat of a chair.

If you lack balance, place a hand on a chair or the wall.

Avoid raising your arms if you suffer from low or high blood pressure. Keep your arms by your side, place them on your front knee or stretched forward.

Benefits:

Creates flexibility and alignment in the hips, legs, and knees. Keep all the muscles fit.

Opens the hips and stretches the quadriceps.

Helps boost energy.

Activates Samana and Apana vayus and balances the lower 5 chakras.

- Stand with your legs open wide. Turn the right foot out at 90-degree angle so your toes are pointing toward the wall.
- Step the left heel back at a 45-degree angle, grounding the heel firmly.
- Square your hips and face forward as much as possible.
- Rotate the hips back and forth and notice if this brings the hips into a more forward facing position and then hold.
- Avoid overarching your low back by engaging Mulabandha and Uddiyanabandha and letting the sacrum down.

- Press the back heel into the floor and bend the front knee at a 90-degree angle so the knee is right on top of the ankle.
- Lift your arms up in front of the body and overhead, lock your fingers and place them behind the head.
- Press the head and neck back into the hands, to align the head over the torso as you drop the shoulder blades down the back.
- Extend your arms up. Keep your little fingers hands turned slightly in to create space in the upper back.
- If your shoulders move up towards the ears, separate the arms so the shoulders can be in a neutral position.
- Lengthen your neck in alignment with the spine, gaze softly forward, with your chin parallel to the floor.
- Breathe normally and with each exhalation, let the energy radiate to your body.
- Come back to the center, rest for a moment and then repeat to the other side.

WARRIOR POSE II
(VIRABHADRASANA II)

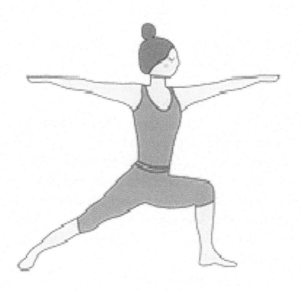

Caution:

If you have weak knees or pain, press the front knee into a folded blanket on the seat of a chair.

For hips problems, use a strap to form a loop from the back heel to the front hip.

If in pain, take a shorter stance, keep the back of your hand on the back hip, or don't do it.

Benefits:

Strengthens and aligns the shoulders, legs, pelvis and hips.

If this pose is held for a long time, it gives the ability to stay calm under pressure.

Works on Samana and Apana vayus, and balances the lower 2 chakras.

- Stand with your legs open wide. Turn the right foot out at a 90-degree angle.
- Turn the left heel at a 30 to 45-degree angle, so your front heel is aligned with the back arch.
- Lift the kneecaps up, and engage Mulabandha and Uddiyanabandha to stabilize the pelvis.
- Lift your arms up to shoulder height and stretch the fingertips in different directions. Gently press the upper arms in the shoulder joints against the stretching of the arms out.
- Move your shoulders down away from the ears, and the shoulder blades down your back.
- Turn your palms up to the ceiling, and while holding the position of the shoulders and upper arms, turn them down again.
- Bend the right knee directly over the right ankle, so that your thigh is parallel to the floor and your knee is right above the ankle.

- Let the hip come down to maintain the alignment of the front knee and ankle.
- Your spine is perpendicular to the floor. Release the sacrum down and gently draw the abdomen in.
- Turn the head looking over the middle finger of the front hand while lifting your crown.
- Breathe normally and with each exhalation let the energy radiate to your body.
- Come back to the center, rest for a moment and then repeat to the other side.

ANNEX 1 – AUTOIMMUNE DISEASES

OUR BODIES HAVE an immune system that is a network of cells and organs that defends the body from foreign invaders like germs. Diseases of the immune system are called autoimmune diseases.

Who gets autoimmune diseases?

According to Women's Health, the people who are at greater risk include:

Young Women — more women than men have autoimmune diseases, and it often starts during their childbearing years.

People with a family history — some autoimmune diseases run in families. Inheriting certain genes can make it more likely to get an autoimmune disease, but a grouping of genes and other factors may cause the disease.

People who are around certain things in the environment such as sunlight, solvents, and viral and bacterial infections, which are linked to many autoimmune diseases.

People of certain ethnic backgrounds — some autoimmune

diseases are more common or touch certain groups of people relentlessly. Type 1 diabetes is common in white people, while Lupus is most severe for African-American and Hispanic people.

What autoimmune diseases affect women, and what are the symptoms?

Many autoimmune diseases share symptoms such as fatigue, light-headedness, and low-grade fever. The symptoms come and go, are sometimes mild and other times severe, and can disappear for a while or break out unpredictably.

Autoimmune hepatitis – The immune system attacks and destroys the liver cells. Some of the symptoms are fatigue, enlarged liver, yellowing of the skin or whites of eyes, itchy skin, joint pain and stomach upset.

Celiac disease – A disease in which people cannot tolerate gluten, a substance found in wheat, rye, and barley, or some medicines. Some of the symptoms are abdominal bloating and pain, diarrhea or constipation, weight loss or weight gain, fatigue, missed menstrual periods, and itchy skin rash.

Diabetes type 1 – The immune system attacks the cells that make insulin, a hormone needed to control blood sugar levels. Without insulin, too much sugar stays in the blood. High blood sugar can hurt the eyes, kidneys, nerves, and gums and teeth. But the most serious problem caused by diabetes is heart disease. Some of the symptoms are being thirsty, urinating often, feeling hungry or tired, losing weight without trying, dry and itchy skin, or having blurry eyesight.

Graves' disease (hyperthyroid) – The thyroid to make too much thyroid hormone. The symptoms are insomnia, irritability, weight loss, heat sensitivity, sweating, muscle weakness, bulging eyes, and shaky hands. Sometimes there are no symptoms.

Hashimoto's disease (hypothyroid) – The thyroid does not make enough thyroid hormone. The symptoms are fatigue, weakness, weight gain, sensitivity to cold, muscle aches and stiff joints, facial swelling, or constipation.

Inflammatory bowel disease (IBD) – A disease that causes chronic inflammation of the digestive tract. Crohn's disease and ulcerative colitis are the most common forms of IBD. The symptoms are abdominal pain, diarrhea.

Multiple sclerosis (MS) – The immune system attacks the protective coating around the nerves. The damage affects the brain and spinal cord. The symptoms are weakness and trouble with balance, speaking and walking, paralysis, tremors, numbness and tingling feeling in arms, legs, hands, and feet.

Psoriasis – New skin cells that grow deep in your skin rise too fast and pile up on the skin surface. The symptoms are thick red patches covered with scales, usually on the head, elbows, and knees, itching and pain that can make it difficult to sleep or walk. May have a form of arthritis that often affects the joints and the ends of the fingers and toes.

Rheumatoid Arthritis – The immune system attacks the lining of the joints throughout the body. The symptoms are painful, stiff, swollen, and deformed joints, reduced movement and function. May have fatigue, fever, weight loss, eye inflammation, lung disease, and lumps of tissue under the skin.

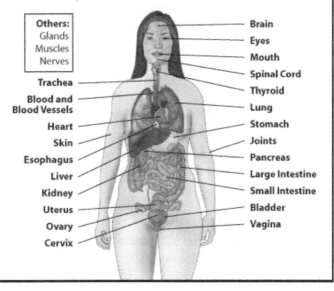

Body Parts That Can Be Affected by Autoimmune Diseases

Others:
Glands
Muscles
Nerves

Trachea
Blood and Blood Vessels
Heart
Skin
Esophagus
Liver
Kidney
Uterus
Ovary
Cervix

Brain
Eyes
Mouth
Spinal Cord
Thyroid
Lung
Stomach
Joints
Pancreas
Large Intestine
Small Intestine
Bladder
Vagina

ANNEX 2 – BALANCING THE DOSHAS

ACCORDING TO AYURVEDA, a healthy mind and body is one in which the vital energy forces of Vata, Pita, and Kapha are in harmony.

I strongly recommend the practice of the Joint Freeing Series as designed by Mukunda Stiles in his Structural Yoga Therapy book especially those who have a Vata imbalance. It has helped me tremendously in managing fatigue and aching muscles.

VATA

The following practices are recommended to bring Vata into balance:

- Practicing regularly the Joint Freeing Series.
- Standing poses to give strength to the base of the body.
- Balancing poses to increase strength and stability.
- Heat-building poses.
- Holding the poses for longer time.

- Using props such as blocks, bolsters, foam wedges, or a wall for support.
- Focusing on regular and mindful breathing in the poses.

PITTA

The following practices are recommended to bring Pitta into balance:

- Standing poses that emphasize hip opening.
- Cooling poses.
- Calming poses while avoiding extra effort.
- Rapid sun salutations.
- Taking time between poses to realize the benefit(s) of each pose.
- Focusing on the exhalation.

KAPHA

The following practices are recommended to bring Kapha into balance:

- Standing poses and back-bend to create heat and energy while opening the chest.
- Inverted poses that require effort and induce a new perspective.
- Mindful movement to start a pose when done by itself or as part of a flow.
- Focusing on the inhalation and the upward drive of energy.

ANNEX 3 – SEQUENCE FOR RHEUMATOID ARTHRITIS

Y<small>OU CAN DO</small> this practice at the opening of yoga practice. It helps in releasing excessive wind and acid from the body, mainly the joints. You can sit on a chair, a mat or a blanket.

This sequence is at a beginner level and beneficial for all age groups. Anyone with good health can practice it. Mindfully coordinate these movements of the various joints with your breathing and you will reap many benefits.

Focus on stretching and flexing the various joints in the body, including the muscles, creating space for smooth flow of prana as you work on removing blocked passages.

Breathe normally while practicing.

1. Relaxation pose (Savasana) for 1 minute.
2. Staff pose (Dandasana) for 30 seconds.
3. Extend your legs forward, point your toes then curl them. Repeat for 40 seconds.
4. Rotate your ankles one way then the other way for 40 seconds.

5. Sit on a chair, bend one leg and place the ankle on the other leg. Rotate the ankle one way then another for 40 seconds. Then switch and repeat with the other leg.

6. Sit on a chair or blanket, bend your leg placing the ankle on the thigh of the other leg then rotate your knee for 30 seconds. Repeat on the other side.

7. Extend your legs forward. Inhale and lift one leg up, exhale and bend the leg, inhale lift it up again, exhale and lower it down. Do this on both legs for 30 seconds each leg.

8. Sit on a mat or a blanket and bring the soles of your feet together in front and pull them as close to your hips as is comfortable. Let your knees drop out to the side. Keep lifting in your torso without forcing. Hold the outside edge of your feet and let your knees drop out to the sides. Breathe normally for 40 seconds.

9. Clench your hands then extend all your fingers and repeat for 30 seconds.

10. Wrist Bending – extend your arms and bend your hands fingers pointing down then up, and repeat for 30 seconds.

11. Wrist Joint rotation one way then the other way for 40 seconds.

12. Extend your arms forward, bend your elbows so that the fingers touch the shoulders close to the neck then extend them. Repeat for 40 seconds.

13. Shoulder Circles one way then the other way for 40 seconds.

14. Neck Rolls one way then the other way for 40 seconds.

ANNEX 4 – SEQUENCE FOR A HEALTHY CIRCULATORY SYSTEM

FOR A HEALTHY CIRCULATORY SYSTEM, you could do a combination of some of these movements:

- Starting from the Table pose, do cat lifts and rolls, table twist, regular child pose, sunbird, and child pose with elbows crossed hugging the shoulders.
- Starting from a standing position, do the triangle, warrior II, chair, and separate leg forward fold poses.
- While lying down on your back, do the knee-to-chest pose, pelvic tilt, followed by the bridge poses.
- Lying on your abdomen, do the locust, sphinx, cobra, downward dog, and plank poses.
- From a seated position, do the legs up the wall, spinal twist, head to knee, forward bend, cow's head, and staff poses.
- Visualizations – Bring the breath gently into your heart centre. As you exhale, let the tension flow away from the heart. As you inhale feel totally relaxed. Find a place in your body that feels most relaxed and bring that energy into your heart centre.

- Relaxation for 5 to 10 minutes.

ANNEX 5 – MOVEMENTS TO AVOID BASED ON AUTOIMMUNE CONDITION

- Abdominal pain (from IBS or Celiac disease) – Stay away from flexion, rotation and any spinal movement that worsens pain.
- Anxiety – Stay away from backbends if the symptoms are active.
- Back pain – Adjust movements of the spine that cause pain and use caution for flexion and extension.
- Degenerative disc of the spine – Stay away from movement that cause pain and spine flexion. Flexion of the spine is when you bring the front of your torso close to your legs.
- Diabetes – Avoid deep spinal twists, full inversions. If it's Diabetes Type 1, avoid full inversions.
- Fibromyalgia – Stay away from movement that causes pain.
- High blood pressure – Stay away from inversions and long hold of standing poses. Inverting is when you go upside down, even in part, and your heart is higher than your head.

- Irritable Bowel Syndrome – Stay away from deep spinal twist or flexion that worsens symptoms.
- Multiple Sclerosis – Stay away from overheating. Do only gentle movements of joints.
- Osteoarthritis – Stay away from weight-bearing movement at any joint that has arthritic pain.
- Osteoporosis – Stay away from flexion of spine, and be careful when you rotate the spine deeply.
- Spondylolisthesis of spine – Stay away from extension of spine and check with your orthopedic doctor for more contraindications.

ANNEX 6 – BALANCING THE VAYUS

THE SOLES of the feet and the crown of the head are linked at both ends of the body. When the breath moves freely between them, we sense the whole body. This helps to be grounded and free.

Caution: Do not force the breath. Let the breath flow smoothly and gently.

Benefits: A general boost and calming. With regular practice, your breath flows steadily, your concentration will improve, and your body will feel reinvigorated.

1. Lie down on a yoga mat or a blanket. For more support, place a small cushion under your head and/or roll up a blanket under your knees.
2. Slowly scan the body from head to toe, relax your mind and let go of tension.
3. Start with a relaxed diaphragmatic breathing. Next,
4. Exhale as if the breath is flowing from the crown of your head down to your toes. Inhale back to the

crown of the head. Repeat 2 or 3 times here and at each consecutive point except when told otherwise.

5. Exhale to your ankles, and inhale back to the crown.

6. Exhale to your knees, and inhale back to the crown.

7. Exhale to the base of your spine, and inhale back to the crown.

8. Exhale to your navel center, and inhale back to the crown.

9. Exhale to your heart center, and inhale back to the crown.

10. Exhale to your throat, and inhale back to the crown.

11. Exhale to your eyebrow center. Breathe back and forth between the crown and your eyebrow center 5 to 10 times, to refine the breath.

12. Now reverse the order and come down, first to the throat center, then to the heart center, to the navel center, and so on, until you return to the toes.

13. Finish by breathing as if the whole body breathes.

14. Gradually bend the knees and slowly roll unto your side.

15. Resting on your side for a few moments, become conscious of the effects of the practice.

16. Press yourself upright to a seated position. Stay for a moment with your hands at your heart bowing to your higher self and to the practice you just did.

ANNEX 7 – SEQUENCE FOR DIABETES

DIABETES MAY NOT HAVE a complete cure, but diabetic people can take steps to manage or control their blood sugar.

Blood glucose or blood sugar is a key source of energy and comes from the food we eat and digest. Diabetes happen when the blood glucose is too high or too low. Insulin, a hormone made by the pancreas, helps transform the glucose we get from food to be used for energy. At times, the body does not make any or enough insulin or does not use it properly. The glucose then stays in the blood without getting to the cells. This produces excess glucose in the blood, which causes some health problems.

Common kinds of diabetes are:

Type 1–the body does not make enough insulin, the immune system attacks and destroys the cells in the pancreas that is responsible for making insulin.

Type 2–the body does not use the insulin well and glucose is an excess in the blood.

Type 3–Gestational diabetes usually develop in some pregnant women.

This yoga sequence for diabetes targets the digestive system. The poses aim to improve its functioning to an optimal level. Breathe normally while you do these poses.

Easy Pose – 10 to 12 breaths

Caution: Patients with diabetes must keep fruit juice within reach. Seek help and guidance from a medical professional or a yoga therapist when practicing yoga.

Benefits: Calms the body and the mind.

- Sit at the center of a mat, on a cushion or a blanket. Cross your legs comfortably, lift the spine and close your eyes.
- Breathe normally.
- Notice the slow expansion and contraction of the abdomen as you inhale and exhale. Connect with this movement and relax your mind and the muscles of your face.
- Hold this pose for 10 to 12 breaths or more until you feel comfortable with the breath and the body.

Staff Pose (Dandasana) – 6 to 8 breaths

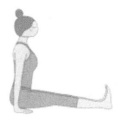

Seated Forward Bend Pose (Paschimottanasana) 6 to 8 breaths

This pose targets the digestive system and the abdominal organs. The stretch is done gently and gradually without forcing. Hold the pose comfortably and avoid going beyond your limits.

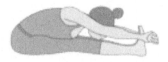

Variation:

- From a seated position, bend the right leg at the knee and have it folded on the floor.
- Bring the right foot close to the perineum (the surface region between the pubic bone and the coccyx) while extending the left leg forward.
- Inhale and raise your arms above your head – or in front of you if you have high blood pressure. As you exhale bring your torso forward and lower your arms to rest your hands on your left shin. Your face is close to your left thigh as much as comfortable.
- Hold this pose for about 4 to 6 breaths making sure that the stretch is gentle. Note if you feel the stretch at the lower back and/or the hamstrings (group of

muscles and their tendons at the back of the upper leg).

- Release the right leg and extend it close to the left leg.
- Repeat on the other leg.
- Gradually, hold the pose a little longer as it has a beneficial effect on the digestive system.

Half Lord of the Fishes Pose Variation Hand Down—4 to 6 breaths

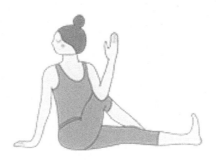

Relaxation Pose—5 to 10 minutes

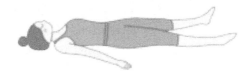

Wind Release Pose–6 to 8 breaths

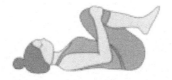

BOOKS, MANUALS AND ARTICLES CONSULTED

H<small>ATHA</small> <small>AND</small> R<small>AJA</small> Y<small>OGA</small> S<small>TUDIES</small> teacher training course–Marie Paulyn.

Yoga Therapy Foundation Program with the Breathing Deeply Yoga Therapy School–Brandt Passalacqua.

Structural Yoga Therapy Adapting to the Individual–Mukunda Stiles.

Integrative Yoga Therapy Yoga Teachers' Toolbox (pages 3-5)–Joseph and Lillian LePage.

Integrative Yoga Therapy Home Study Program (pages 3.17-3.18 of the manual)–Joseph and Lillian LePage.

Women's Health Government site, Office on Women's Health, U.S. Department of Health and Human Services (site visited on March 29, 2019).

Pain Assessment and Management–Toronto Public Library instructor-facilitated online learning.

"Can Yoga Help Curb Chronic Inflammation? New Light on

Disease Prevention" article published in the YogaU online magazine–Lynn Crimando.

Yoga for Healthy Aging - A Guide to Lifelong Well-Being, December 12, 2017–Baxter Bell, MD and Nina Zolotow (pages 291-297).

"Relaxation Practice to Balance the 5 Prana Vayus" article published in the Yoga International online magazine.

ABOUT THE AUTHOR

Liliane Najm, CYA-RYT300

CYA stands for Canadian Yoga Alliance. RYT300 stands for Registered Yoga Teacher 300 hours.

I graduated as a certified teacher of Hatha Yoga with the *School of Hatha and Raja Yoga Studies* in Toronto in 2002. I completed a *Meditation Teacher* training with the OM-Line Yoga and Ayurveda in December 2018; *Yoga for Seniors* with Breathe Yoga Studio in October 2018; and a *Core Confidence Specialist* with Bellies Inc. in July 2018. I am also a Reiki Master/Teacher.

While holding a full-time administration job in downtown Toronto, I am taking the Yoga Wellness Educator training with YogaU. My favourite hobby is writing. Please visit my blog at www.lilianenajm.wordpress.com and leave comments; I will be glad to read them.

I like helping others to achieve healing and wellness through the sciences of yoga practice, mindful movement, breathing techniques, and meditation.

Send me an email if you have a question about this eBook. You can reach me at liliane_najm@yahoo.ca.

Made in the USA
Las Vegas, NV
18 January 2022

41791127R00108